Dear Pete,

What's Next Papa was written by Pat's grand-nephew, Scott Roix. NSCBC prayed for him and his family during that very difficult time the book details.

WHAT'S NEXT, PAPA?

"Papa" is Scott's special name for God. His wife, Nette, whom we had met, wrote a blog throughout and inspired us and really made us think about life and its hard times. This is a story of deep sadness but also ultimate victory through the strength God gives when hard things come to us. Her passing was difficult for all who knew her, but she is now with "Papa." God was with Scott and Nette throughout their struggle. It's about real life — but also about God's amazing grace.

May God become even more so, "Papa" to you by reading this book.

Peter (dictated)

WHAT'S NEXT, PAPA?

A Story of Cancer that Awakened Hope and Brought Life

S. R. Roix

iUniverse, Inc.
Bloomington

WHAT'S NEXT, PAPA?
A Story of Cancer that Awakened Hope and Brought Life

iUniverse books may be ordered through booksellers or by contacting:

iUniverse
1663 Liberty Drive
Bloomington, IN 47403
www.iuniverse.com
1-800-Authors (1-800-288-4677)

Because of the dynamic nature of the Internet, any web addresses or links contained in this book may have changed since publication and may no longer be valid. The views expressed in this work are solely those of the author and do not necessarily reflect the views of the publisher, and the publisher hereby disclaims any responsibility for them.

Any people depicted in stock imagery provided by Thinkstock are models, and such images are being used for illustrative purposes only.
Certain stock imagery © Thinkstock.

ISBN: 978-1-4620-5328-5 (sc)
ISBN: 978-1-4620-5329-2 (hc)
ISBN: 978-1-4620-5330-8 (ebk)

Library of Congress Control Number: 2011916846

Printed in the United States of America

iUniverse rev. date: 10/06/2011

CONTENTS

ACKNOWLEDGMENTS

Writing a book has been an experience that is way beyond my expertise. That is putting it mildly. I am very grateful to all who have participated with me helping to bring this memoir to a published book. To my good friends Don and Janet Maxon—Without your persistent questioning of how the writing was going, I probably never would have started. Thank you for keeping it before me.

To my new mom-in-law, Grandma Candy—Yours was the unenviable task of reading the scratches I made on paper and translating them into intelligible words on a computer. You are the best. Thank you.

To my wife, Gina—What an amazing gift you have given me. Without your support for this project I never would have been able to move forward with the writing. I appreciate *every* painstaking minute you put into making of this book. I know it was not an easy read for you. You are a great companion.

Brandon and Tracy—Just like Grandma Candy had the difficult job of reading my handwriting, you, too, had the painstaking task of interpreting my thoughts and then making them readable. It seems I did not pay very close attention in grammar class. Thank you for your diligence.

Thank you to my family. I am a very wealthy man because of each of you in my life. Thank you for your support as I read and then reread the manuscript aloud to you.

Finally, thank you to my God. Without God there would be no story to share. The tale would have gone much differently had it not been for Your closeness and constant reassurance. No matter how bleak the path may have looked, You were with me. From the core of who I am I cry with a loud voice . . . *THANK YOU!*

PROLOGUE

God speaks to His children. There's no doubt about it. His voice is distinct and His messages are clear. The question is, "Can you hear Him?"

If you had asked Scott Roix this question a few years ago, he would have answered, "Yes," looking all the way back to his youth in Northern Maine and up until he settled with his young family in Ottawa, Illinois. This was the truth because he did know how to hear God speak.

Today, if you ask Scott this same question you will discover that his answer is still "Yes," but it only takes a few moments to realize that this "Yes" is quite different than the first one. He now knows that God is speaking to him constantly and that he can enjoy a depth of fellowship with *Papa* that he never knew was possible before the incidents he writes about in this book.

In a few moments you will begin reading Scott's story, discovering that there is a practical connection between the stories of Abraham, David, Gideon, Moses, and others with the pathway God chose for Scott Roix. Like these Bible giants, Scott has learned to depend upon God through a crisis of faith that touched every area of his life.

Over this past year it has been my privilege to meet with Scott on a weekly basis in a coaching relationship. During these times I've seen the intensity of Scott's love for God and his determination to use every moment of his life to leave a Kingdom impact with his family, his church, and his world.

You will be greatly encouraged by each chapter and each story Scott tells in this book. You'll soon see that he has been seeking God's face as he has read God's Word, as he has worshiped God, and as he has experienced each of life's situations. He has learned to see God's fingerprints in each one.

Ask God to help you learn as Scott has that when it comes to life, "I am not the author. God is!" Learning this lesson will cause you to ask, *"What's Next Papa?"*

> Don Robins
> Senior Pastor
> Harvest Community Church
> Oak Creek, Wisconsin
> November, 2010

INTRODUCTION

The Call

Recently, I had the opportunity to attend an awards banquet. The presenter for the evening opened with the telling of his recent health scare. I don't recall many details of his story; however, one part did grab my attention—it was his reliving "the call" he received from his doctor. The man replayed the moments of terror that went through his mind as the physician delivered the life-altering news. He told the audience how nothing else mattered at that moment . . . everything came to a halt. Whatever was on his calendar instantly became unimportant. This was the matter of life and death. A realization settled in that his life would not last forever.

I have thought of his story often. I, to, know what it is like to answer the phone and have news that forever alters life's course. The "call" was not for me; it was for my 38 year old wife and mother of our four children. The doctor's report was renal cell carcinoma. The world stopped at that moment: **CANCER.** My mind was already playing the tape of days that had yet to be lived. None of my imagined scenarios ended with, " . . . and they lived happily ever after." No, my imagination took the darker path of grief, death, and loss. Even now, three plus years removed from that phone conversation, I recall with vivid detail the deep sense of despair that instantly washed over me. Helpless! How could this be true? She is so young, so full of life, and has so much to live for.

The doctor's call was not for me that day; it was for my wife, Annette. However, I too had a call. Mine was of a different sort. I have come to speak of my call as Job's choice. Job, a book from the Old Testament, is the story of how this man of antiquity faced some of the most devastating, gut wrenching news anyone could hear . . . one after another. Sitting in the ruins of a once familiar life his wife came and offered the suggestion that Job should just get it over: "Curse God and die." (Job 2:9) He did not take her advice but instead chose to trust that God knew and cared about him and what was going on in his life. That has been my call: trust God.

I did not understand what purpose a young wife and mother being diagnosed with cancer could possibly serve. I still don't understand it; but this I know—God called me to trust Him no matter the outcome.

I wrote this book as a story of hope for anyone who might have just received "the call." Your world has crashed to the ground. In the first several chapters I record stories from Scripture of men who chose to trust God in the most ridiculous ways. Stories that give a framework to better understand my own circumstances. Perhaps, like the stories I have recorded, it seems insane to trust that God is in control. I admit most times it feels more natural, perhaps even the first response, to do as Job's wife suggested, "Curse God." If HE really is good and loving, then why is this happening to me, why my family?

My plea to you is to hold off cursing. Try crying out to God instead—often, He is found in the middle of intense pain. I think you will find, like the stories from Scripture and from my own experience, that God is involved in every detail. I would love to hear how "Papa" walked with you in life's darkest hours.

CHAPTER 1

A Look Back

I left my childhood home of northern Maine in the fall of 1990 to enroll in a small Christian college in Dover, Delaware. The very first day I was there, while still unpacking, I looked out the window and saw her. I was absolutely taken. She was beautiful! It has been a tendency of mine to go headlong into something and my pursuit of Annette K. Stanfield was no different. Nette, a popular third year student who had a large network of friends, I, on the other hand, didn't. I was mostly there on my own with only a few acquaintances from Maine. I began the quest to find out who this girl was. At night, my roommate would hammer at my vulnerability informing me that there was no way she would ever notice me. I knew he was right, my thoughts about myself were anything but favorable. I felt like a nerd; I had extremely thick glasses that magnified my eyes to the size of saucers and at twenty years old, already had a receding hairline. In spite of my insecurities, I somehow won her affection.

The college we attended had very strict guidelines for first year students regarding dating. As I think about it . . . they had strict guidelines about everything! One of the policies was that new students were not allowed to date until Christmas banquet. That was our first "official" date. Already there were feelings that the relationship had potential beyond casual dating. So the timeline goes: met for the first time in August, first date in December, married the

1

following August. I only offer a sketch of the next fifteen-plus years, leading up to the main point of my writing.

Upon completion of my studies at Kent Christian College, we accepted the offer to work with the youth at Annette's uncle's church. Freshly graduated from a two year Biblical studies course, we were eager for the chance to implement our training. When we arrived in Ottawa, Illinois, we did not know what was stirring just below the surface. The pastor belonged to an organization that was applying pressure to its members to hold a more strict interpretation of Scripture.

Within a year of being in our new surroundings, the whole religious landscape changed. The college, from which I had recently graduated, was also a part of the religious tradition that I had grown up in. Everything I knew of God was viewed through that lens. These were unsettling days. It felt as though my whole foundation of faith was being shaken. There was no way of knowing it was the first of many tests. I vividly recall a church service during that time. The speaker was being obnoxious, in my opinion; I left my seat and headed for the door. My pastor was close behind. "What's going on?" he inquired. My response was that I didn't know if there was a God . . . and I really didn't care. That was not true! I cared more than anything. I wanted to know Him! I wanted to know more than anything that He was true. Even though I held a degree in Biblical Studies, it appeared that I did not have a clue whom God was. In that discouraged mindset I laid down any thought of "ministry." I did not know the answers for myself, how could I expect to point anyone else in the right direction?

I began working construction with Annette's family and did so for the next seven years. Life began to have a rhythm to it. We had two children during that season and began to settle into familiar routines. All was well—so it appeared. Cracks were beginning to form in Annette's veneer; you know, the exterior that you try to portray to everyone that everything is fine/I'm okay/can't you see my smile? The reality was that she felt close to having a breakdown.

One of the cornerstones of our relationship was our ability to communicate with each other. Annette joined a group of women from our church attending a weekend retreat a few hours from our home. It was around 8 o'clock on Sunday evening when she returned. When Nette walked in she announced we needed to talk—sometime. I felt there was no better time than right *now*. Over the next several hours, I heard things that sent me reeling. It felt as if a professional boxer had taken his best shot to my unguarded solar plexus. The air was completely knocked from me. My wife began telling me how several people had sexually abused her from an early age. She was recalling places . . . times . . . things in the room . . . smell—on and on. Later, after months of counseling she was able to put her finger on a simple phrase that was told to her as a young child: you have nothing I want. She would come to say that those five words set the course for her life.

She often thought of herself as a prostitute as she would try to disprove those words that had been planted in her mind. The stories that came pouring out held incredible shame for her; they had an opposite effect on me. She thought that if anyone really knew who she was . . . really knew the filth that she had been dragged through . . . she would be rejected, an outcast. That is why it was easier to adopt the "I'm okay" look. That can only last for so long before the truth begins to seep through the cracks. What Nette found, to her amazement, was not rejection. She found people who loved her . . . people who were the arms of God with their embrace. She found words that gave life . . . words from people that Nette loved and respected. She found that I did not want to leave her, as her thoughts had been informing her. I did not look at her as a prostitute. What I did next was not to say, "Look at how great I am," but rather to say "Look how loving God is."

I had a desire to marry my wife again. This time I would marry her with full knowledge of who she was—scars and all. It was in this season that the story of Hosea became so poignant in Nette's life. God told the prophet that He was going to show Israel an object lesson of how much He loved them. Hosea was to marry a prostitute and repeatedly go after her and bring her home. Show her love—true love . . . beautiful love. I did not think of Nette in terms of a prostitute; that was a label she had given herself. I know God used me to bring healing to one of His beautiful daughters who had been so mistreated.

I cannot report at this point in the story that Annette was completely healed of her past. I can say that she began to heal by degrees for years to come. It was in this atmosphere of new beginnings that we decided to have a child. We gave the name Karrigan to our new baby girl. Our pastor gave a masterful use of words at her dedication back to God. He spoke to Nette directly and prayed that every time she called out the name of our daughter she would "Care-Again."

I pause from the telling of my story and write to those who are holding onto secrets . . . secrets that are informing you about who you are—or are *not*; secrets that are toxic—with an end result that is not very appealing. The Bible says that there is indeed an enemy. This enemy comes to steal . . . kill . . . and destroy. If this power of darkness can get an individual to hold onto a secret and have no one be able to speak truth to that darkness: Enemy—1, Victim—0. You lose! But if you find a safe place: a counselor, friend, spouse, pastor—someone you know who loves you—I encourage you: *get it out into the light.* Enough of letting those thoughts that can be all consuming control your life. I am not a professional counselor, by any means . . . I have lived through it! I only speak with experience. I saw how destructive those thoughts could be and I also witnessed the unwavering truth of Scripture. 2 Kings puts it this way: *"Choose life and not death" (18:32).* You will need to make the deliberate decision to move your feet up those stairs, open the door, and begin forming words about your story. It can be terrifying; it takes a huge amount of courage; it is worth it!

The next several years blur together—family growing in age, and in size. We had an unexpected gift in the form of Zachary. I have often joked that our kids' names are Lo-Gan, Meg-Gan, Karri-Gan, and finally . . . Not-a-Gan. We didn't have the nerve to name him that, but we did break the rhyme and called him Zachary.

I joined an electrical union, Nette homeschooled our children for several years. We were doing okay. I was making the most money ever in my life; we were able to do most things that we always wanted to do. At one point I read a book that inspired me to buy rental property and managed to lose a few more hair follicles. There is a book in the telling of those stories. I leave it at: I am not cut out to own rental property!

Life was good. If I were to finish the story of where the Roix family was headed, it would have had kids growing up, heading off to college, beginning their own lives, bringing over the grandkids . . . meanwhile, Nette and I would travel for both mission and leisure. But—I am not the author. God is! God is the One Who knows the number of our days. And, as we were about to learn . . . those days are not without end.

The words on the pages that you are about to read record some of the darkest, loneliest, disorienting days of my life. I never dreamt it would happen to me . . . not to *my* family . . . not *my* children.

CHAPTER 2

Walking by Faith

Thrilling, terrifying, *God, I want it more than anything* (what in the world am I doing): **Walking by faith**. Lately I'd been reading the account of Abraham. I had been viewing stories and characters in the Bible with a new perspective that I had never before considered. For some reason, I'd read the stories numerous times with the thought that the characters in the stories knew the outcomes already. It's probably common to think that way: "Well, you know, that was *Abraham* . . . or the superstar, *Noah*; they had an inside track with God. When He spoke to them they knew it was going to happen." I can only imagine what Abraham's conversation with God must have looked like:

Abraham is going about his business and Genesis says God showed up and spoke to him. Something along the lines of giving Abraham so many descendants they would be numbered like sand, as numerous as stars. God continued to tell this ninety-nine year old man the terms of the blessing: he has to go home and take a sharp stone and circumcise every male in his house! Anyone with a Webster's dictionary and a good imagination knows that it is not a pleasant afternoon at the Abraham residence for the male gender.

Hello! Not sure it is God talking anymore. Imagine the conversation when Abraham comes back to 1805 Tent Ave.

"Hey, Sarah, I had a visitor today. It was God! He told me we were going to have a lot of children . . . No, really. He said they would be numbered as many as there are grains of sand."

No wonder Sarah laughed. She is in her nineties, her husband nearing the century mark: not exactly *People* magazine cover material.

Even though his wife is rolling on the floor, thinking that the old guy has gone mad, Abraham continues. "Yeah, He said we are going to have a child a year from now and He wanted to make a contract with me. I am to take a sharp stone and cut off the foreskin of every male in our house. That way we are marked as His."

Now, the way I had read this story in the past was, of course, that Abraham, his teenage son Ishmael, his servants . . . *all* the guys jockeyed for position at the front of the assembly line. No question! As I mentioned, my thinking has had a shift. I'm guessing from Sarah's response of laughter at the thought of the geriatric birthing of a nation that Abraham's family was a little skeptical of Abraham's lunch appointment, especially the male gender!

The stories go on and on like that. Noah builds a gigantic vessel that holds enough animals to keep the species going . . . even though it had never before rained. What must the neighbors have thought? "He is nuts!" Gideon, leading an army that is already vastly outnumbered by a powerful enemy, reduces his force to only a handful after an encounter with God. Joshua, another one of scripture's crazies, gathers his leaders to inform them that God let him in on a plan of how to destroy an enemy city:

"Okay guys, here's what we are going to do!" (I picture a huddle of middle-aged men playing football on a Sunday afternoon).

"Guys, we're going to walk around this enormous wall once a day for six days. On the seventh day we're going to make seven laps, and . . . listen to this . . . here is the good part: on my mark, everybody yell as loud as you can, break your jars and blow your trumpets!"

That's what God said. Yikes! What kind of plan is that? Wonder what I would have had to say if I had been in that huddle? "Well, you know, Joshua that might be a fine plan, but what if we try this first?" Then I would try my best to get this nut job to do something a little more conventional and not cause a whole group of people to look like a circus freak show while being annihilated.

Story after story, book after book, God continues to say—and *do*—the ridiculous. Here's another case that baffles me. Imagine this scene:

Hosea . . . today, we call him a prophet. Not sure everyone among his contemporaries gave him the same title. He hears God say to *marry a prostitute*. Seems God wanted to send a message to the Israelite nation by giving them an object lesson. The prophet Hosea hears that he is to marry a lady of the night. Mmmhmm . . . *sure* . . . that's what God said. I've worked with a guy who dated a stripper. If he had come to work saying it was God who said to do it, well, I would have had another label for him. It would not have been *prophet.*

Each of these men of ancient times *believed*. They were unsophisticated enough to do what God asked them to do. I tell myself that was then and this is now. We are much more enlightened than they were. It's just different . . . we have iPads now.

In each of the stories to which I refer, I can hear my own voice in the crowd. It is often on the side of those ridiculing the one who reports, "God said." I can imagine if I'd sat in the circle as Abraham gathered his family around to fill them in on God's plan to make a great nation from their clan. What if I were a bystander as Noah begin gathering materials in preparation to build a boat after "hearing" God lay out the plan to destroy the earth by flooding it.

What if someone were to have a visit like that today? My skepticism would be on high alert. It all seems too unbelievable . . . impossible . . . improbable. Why would God interact with humans to clue them in on His activity?

My mind has been traveling to these places of late as a result of where the journey, called life, has been taking me. Twists and bends along the path have delivered me to a place where I, too, like the stories I have written about, have a choice: trust and live the impossible, or . . . turn on my heel and reject any notion that God is involved in any way.

The past year and a half have delivered me to Christ. I have often read the Bible as an obligation . . . a duty: if you call yourself a Christian, you should do this. Yeah, it may be tedious and somewhat irrelevant to my 21st-century life, but I must do it in order to check it off my to-do list of being a "good Christian." But now, like the man named Job in the oldest writing of the Bible, in the famous story of suffering, he reports at the end of his experience, and I paraphrase, that he had heard hearsay of God, but now, *now*, after all he'd been through . . ."*Now I know him.*" My own passage through grief has given me a similar perspective.

Before this past year's struggles, my faith was something of a theory with a few experiences along the way that kind of kept it interesting enough to keep going. I have always had a hunger for God. Jesus preached (Matthew 5:6), "*You're blessed when you've worked up a good appetite for God. He's food and drink in the best meal you'll ever eat.*" I can read that and it doesn't even register. "Best meal you ever tasted," . . . *okay*, a little hyperbole going on; I have had some very good meals and I'm not so sure God had anything to do with it. Yet, still, I wanted to experience it. Could that, and a thousand other verses, actually be true? Is it really possible to "taste" of God . . . and find it to be "the best meal I have ever tasted?" Oh, how I want that to be true. I want all of it to be true.

Another verse that grabs me is written in Mark 6:12 where Jesus sent His followers out and *"They preached with a joyful urgency that life could be radically different."* Wow! That staggers me. My generalization of the western church is that we are not radically different from those who do not believe in Christ. Do I think that following Him is indeed the very best way to live? Has my own life been "radically" affected as a result of following this man called Christ? There would have been a day when I could not have answered "yes" truthfully, but today I can.

Mark, one of the first followers of Christ, tells a story about the men who were on the boat with Jesus when a storm came up. They were so afraid! I know the feeling: everything swirling around my life points to my demise. Waves coming over the bow, ropes on the sail are whipping about in chaos. The boat leans over at a 30ᵈ angle, threatening to toss its occupants overboard. Oh—I forgot—Jesus is right there . . . *sleeping*!! How did I not remember that He was on the boat? For some reason my senses are at code red concerning all of my surroundings: Look at the towering wave of being unemployed, the menacing wind of how to provide for a family of eleven. Everything, EVERYTHING, I see with such clarity. Why, then, can I not see Jesus in the stern of the boat . . . sleeping . . . *unconcerned* about the surface activities. He *trusts*!!

He knows who He is and He knows who His father is. Trust—simple, pure, and childlike; trust. Even if it does not go well, even if the boat sinks, even if . . . *He trusts*. My heart longs to learn this lesson. What could He do if we completely, with abandon, *trust*? It might not look successful according to western culture's standard of success. It could look quite scary, actually! Christ Himself wasn't a sterling model of success: preached for three years, ended up being executed, all His followers scattering like scared sheep. If we only had that snapshot of time to judge His life, it was a total failure.

The story wasn't finished.

Neither is yours—or mine.

It beckons to the adventurer . . .

Where can He take me?

CHAPTER 3

He Loves Me

In Luke 15, Jesus is telling stories, like He often did. He gives His audience three examples of how important it is to Him that those who are lost be found. The first is a story of a shepherd who had a hundred sheep and one got separated from the flock. It was so important to the shepherd to find the lost sheep that he left ninety-nine of them to go look for the one that was lost. The next example from the Storyteller was about a lady who lost one of her ten coins. The woman was so persistent in her search that she scoured her house looking in every nook and cranny for the one lost coin. The last of the three stories is one of my favorites. Most translations of the Bible call it, "The Return of the Prodigal," or, "The Lost Son Comes Home." I have come to think of it, "A father's costly love for his children." This story so captivates me. One of my favorite lines is when the son is making his way back to his father's house from the place where he became lost. The father sees him while he was still way, way, way down the road. Papa runs to him and lavishes love on his child who is still filthy from living with livestock. The boy begins to deliver his prepared speech but the Bible says, *"The Father wasn't [even] listening"* (Luke 15:22). He wasn't listening because he was too busy giving instructions to his staff on how to prepare the extravagant celebration.

The first time I really noticed this story was when I was leading a discussion group in our home. The group was designed around book studies: one that we came across was a small paperback by Henri Nouwen entitled, *"Return of the Prodigal"*. As we read Nouwen's perspective on the story Christ told, something clicked. Could it really be true that God is not angry with me?!? Was there a remote chance that He might even be excited about me and where I am right now? Not someday when I get my act together, but *today*? He is pleased with me *today*! With all of my stuff—wrong thoughts, ugly attitudes, impatience towards people. Even with the stench lingering from life apart from Him, Papa wanted me in His house! I found that hard to believe. In each story, the one doing the looking is an example of God's posture toward us, His creation. Could it really be true that the One Who made heaven and earth is so interested in me that He, metaphorically speaking, sweeps the house in a frantic search? Or that He is like the father whose son publically humiliated him—each day standing, looking down the road, waiting for the boy to return? And once the son comes into view, acting in such an abnormal way for someone who had been so shunned. He sets up tents for a festival: "My son—who was dead—is alive! Is that really how it is? Can God love me that much, or is it just a cruel joke? I wonder if it is just as difficult for me to believe God loves me and is leading my life as it was for the people in the stories I've read in the Bible. This is what I mean. The Bible is full of historical tales of how mankind has been given the choice to trust God or reject Him as nonsense. I'll use the telling of Israel's exodus from Egypt as an example. Moses, a central figure in the script, lived a life full of twists that could have caused him to detour from who he was created to be had he not continued to trust what God was doing in his life. The story originates in the Old Testament. There is a people group called the Israelites who are being brutally oppressed by the ruler of Egypt. This is not just any group of people; they are the nation God promised Abraham. This promised offspring found themselves enslaved—no relief in sight;

hopeless. God saw their misery, heard their plea for help. It is around this time that we are introduced to Moses.

This man has an intriguing story. He enters earth's drama at the time when the ruler of Egypt called Pharaoh is feeling very threatened by the population explosion among the Hebrew slaves. He is worried enough that he decrees a law that every male Hebrew child two and under should be put to death. That is a paranoid guy!

The story continues. Moses' mom makes a wicker basket and waterproofs it so she can place her infant son in it for safety. There are so many side roads that I could go down as I read these events from Scripture. You would think there had to be a much safer place for a newborn than a woven basket placed into a river filled with crocodiles up to 1500 pounds (according to *Ask.com*). Uhhhh . . . Mom, have you thought about under the bed? There is a very good chance the king is going to get the child, but this plan seems like she might as well have killed the boy herself.

Okay, so he is in the croc-filled river among the shoreline weeds. Scripture says the boy starts to cry. It so happens that the Pharaoh's daughter needed a bath about that same time. She hears the infant and investigates. The princess must not have heard her daddy's order. She lets baby Moses go home to be raised by . . . his own mother. Now mom not only has her baby back, but she is getting paid for feeding him. How about that!

Now, already this seems like too fantastic of a tale. It gets better. The Pharaoh's daughter lets mom finish nursing the child then brings Moses into the palace to be raised. The Israelite boy grows up eating at the table of the very man who had tried to kill him. How do you interpret a life like that? I wonder if the story was ever told to him. Did he have any clue of his purpose? I continue. Here is a slave boy—who, by the way, is not supposed to be alive—living in the luxury of the king's palace. Not as a slave . . . but as an adopted son! It seems that he must have known his roots. The story goes, that on one of his outings he came across an Egyptian abusing a Hebrew slave. Dilemma: lives in the palace . . . eats the king's meals . . . sleeps comfortably . . . has everything he could want; yet, he sees an injustice being done to his people. I feel his turmoil. The text says he looked both ways to be sure no one was watching. He wants to do the right thing . . . but what if it costs him? Is there any reward for doing the "right thing" besides just feeling good?

Well, he found out soon enough. After he stops the abuse by killing the aggressor, his step-dad, who happens to be Pharaoh, finds out. Yeah, he'll show Moses reward. Moses is forced to flee to the desert.

Sometimes that is what it feels like. You do something good and get rewarded by having to flee to a desert. Yuck. What is that about? How can anyone interpret the events of life?

I can only imagine what was going through Moses' mind as he settled into the routine of desert life. Now, instead of sitting around a table with servants filling his plate, he is the one who has to kill, cook, serve, and clean up. What does he tell himself about his story? Saved from certain death—either by king or by nature—grew up in surroundings that most only dream of, and now he finds himself in a desert!

I wonder what he told himself as he trudged along . . . alone . . . in the desert. "Man, wish I could take those 10 minutes back. I could have . . ." Then he would fill in the blank with different scenarios that affected a more positive outcome than the one in which he found himself.

He did what he thought was right. Misunderstood . . . hurt . . . angry. What did he do with all of that? Did he ponder his path, replaying the steps that lead to the desert? How disorienting it must have been. Moses is saved from certain death at birth—only to find that it lands him in a desert, alone. Why? Why bother living all those days if only he is to die alone . . . misunderstood . . . in a desert? Who is in control—anyone? Is it just the randomness of existence as a human? Just endure, it will end, and then . . . nothing? Is that what it is—or is there more? The way I see the story from Exodus is that Moses just kept walking. He did what was in front of him; what else could he do?

The story of this ancient character did not end there. The thing Moses didn't know was that there was still a life filled with adventure of walking with God in front of him. If I were to stop reading at this point in the story, it would be a huge disappointment. But he kept walking. It seems Moses had to endure desert life for nearly forty years—*forty years!* That is a very long time to wrestle with questions. But then, doing what he always does, the mundane tasks of life, day in/day out routine that he had become accustomed to in the desert—the routine was interrupted one day. Something caught his eye. He must not have stopped hoping that there was more to life than just existing . . . in the desert. Scripture says Moses was distracted and turned aside to investigate. As he did, the most improbable, beyond his wildest imagination, thing happened. God spoke! God spoke from a bush, a bush that did not disintegrate from flames. One author's explanation for the story is that it was the result of Moses' taking of a hallucinogenic drug found in desert plants. I can't prove the theory. I can believe that the same God who created the bush can caused it not to be consumed. I'm not sure what was in Moses' heart about his people—not sure if he had grandiose thoughts of leading the slave nation out from the oppression of Pharaoh. Maybe he wasn't thinking of them at all. Could be that it had been long enough that he had closed that chapter of his story and was just living out his days. No matter where Moses' thoughts were, here in front of him was a burning bush that was talking and the voice identified Himself as God.

God had not missed a thing. That causes hope in me as I interpret the events of my story. No matter what, no matter where—no matter! God has had His eye on me. I have His attention. One of the Psalmists wrote in Psalm 139 it does not matter where we find ourselves in this life. He was so confident of God's love that he wrote, " . . . *if I go to the highest heights, God is there; or my bed is made in hell, still, God is with me.*"

I have been at both ends of that spectrum and know how true it is. The story I unfold on the pages ahead holds them both.

I may never be turned aside from my daily routine to investigate a talking bush. Still, I look for the day when the One Who has ordered my steps to this point will speak with me and let me know where it is we will go from here. As I traveled through some of my darkest days, verses from Scripture gave reason for hope—and purpose in this life. One passage was written by Paul in his letter to the church in Rome. He wrote in his letter in Romans, chapter 8:14-15, that after Christ gives someone a new life, *God's Spirit beckons. There are things to do and places to go! It's adventurously expectant, greeting God with a childlike, "What's next, Papa?"* Those words have become a prayer for me. Although life has dealt a severe blow, there remains the childlike question in me, "What's next, Papa?" I'm not asking with any notion that it will be all sunshine and roses. I'm asking in a way that is eager to know where the Father would take me from here. What new sights will we encounter? What way will I see Christ like I have never viewed Him before?

Back to Moses. He's in a desert, alone, tending to his responsibilities. He turns aside to investigate a bush—that *speaks.* Out of that conversation his whole world changed. No longer would he be shepherding a flock of sheep—God had unimaginable plans for this one-time prince-turned-sheep-herder to lead a slave nation to freedom. I wonder how long it took before he began to put the pieces together. Saved from death at birth, raised in Egypt by the king, fled to the desert, leading sheep . . . oh, but there is more to my life. God began to bring clarity. Moses, you are to go to the Pharaoh and say, "Let my people go."

17

Why does God do that? It seems as though He takes pleasure in asking the thing that hits in the most vulnerable place. The story doesn't come out and say it plainly, but it sure indicates how much Moses resisted.

You might think it's enough reason to believe God if you are standing in front of the talking shrub. Nope! Oh, how well I know that feeling. So many, many, many signs point to God's leading of my life—yet when it comes to today, looking into an unknown future . . . short term memory loss sets in.

CHAPTER 4

Anyone Need a Truck?

To this point in the story I have mostly talked about characters from the Bible who did the most unorthodox things. They simply believed what was being asked of them and then did it. I have been considering these stories because my path has felt a little unorthodox. The challenge has been to do as those in Scripture: trust . . . believe . . . hope. It has been the most remarkable, *amazing* ride I have ever taken. I pick up the telling of my story in the winter of 2007.

I had been a foreman for a small electrical company for almost 6 years. It really was a great job. The core group of guys felt like brothers. The owner would often take the foremen to golf outings or to workshops about our craft. Most days it was fun. Plenty of work: [as] a matter of fact, it was during the housing boom of the late 90's—early 2000's. A crew was required to wire anywhere from one to five houses a week. The Nextel phone in my tool pouch was a constant reminder of the load of work to be done. Then it all began to unravel. The housing market slowed down. There wasn't the demand for as many on each crew, the foremen became workers and workers became unemployed. The company began to lose contracts . . . the snowball gained momentum. One day I went to the bank to deposit my weekly payroll check only to have the teller inform me they were no longer accepting checks from my employer. There had been too many returned due to insufficient funds. Well, after the fourth one bouncing, Annette and I decided we had better make other plans for employment. It was a Sunday night and a group of friends from the church we attended had prearranged an informal meeting. The gathering was not intended to spotlight our need, but as the evening went on, we, and the place in which we found ourselves, became the focus. It was a difficult spot. I could stay employed and hope to get paid . . . *someday,* or return to the union hall and sign my name at the end of the line of those who were already out of work. At that point the waiting time to go back to work was being projected at one year. Anxiety! What in the world was I going to do? When your budget is used to an income of X amount of dollars, the thought of being unemployed for a year was terrifying. At night, usually around two in the morning, waves of hand-wringing thoughts began. On and on, the endless loop of thought spiraled down. I got up in the morning exhausted and depressed.

It was in this frame of mind that I found myself on that Sunday night. The leaders began to ask questions so their prayer could be better focused. As we talked more, there was a growing consensus that I should consider starting my own electrical company. I must admit . . . that was the furthest thing from my mind at the beginning of the evening. Conversation swirled with possibilities. I had made numerous contacts throughout the years and was sure my reputation for quality craftsmanship would do me well.

I am still a little surprised how everything that happens is the result of words being spoken—and then acted on. Someone had to say out loud: I think we can go to the moon! Wheels were set in motion to accomplish those words. That's how it happened. That night I went home and went to bed not thinking of how the whole thing was going to corkscrew into the ground; rather, thoughts of what *could* be filled my imagination. The next morning I made the commute to the jobsite and resigned my position. It was still only a theory at that point so I'm sure the men I worked with must have thought

I had gone on a Sunday night binge. I vividly remember the ride home after stopping by the union hall. I felt like I could breathe. Freedom: I now had a plan of action and was about to implement it, as hare-brained as it may have seemed.

Illinois did not offer a state-issued electrical license; everything was done on the local level. I went to city hall and signed up for the next available test. The day of the exam I joined a room full of men trying to pass the first hurdle on my way to opening a new business. If I didn't get the license there would be no purpose in pursuing the rest of the details of building a company. All the electrical experience I had was in residential. The exam had everything on it. Everything! I sat on that chair for six straight hours toiling over each question. Question 15 may have been too difficult but question 72 held a clue that led to the answer. That's how it went! When I finally handed it in I was quite unsure of the outcome. The proctor said we should have the results in a day of two. The next morning a lady I knew from city hall called my cell. "Hi Scott, I know what you got on your test. Would you like to know now or wait until you get it in the mail?" I am not very good at waiting. Christmas is as hard on me as it is the kids. Of course I wanted to know. "You passed," she said. Phew! First hurdle was done.

All this time I was mulling over in my mind what I was going to do about a vehicle for my new business. I thought for a while I would get by with using the family mini-van. I hated that though, I wanted to look professional while driving around our community . . . not like a fly-by-night outfit. It was on Wednesday that I took the test, got the call that I had passed on Thursday and now . . . on to Friday.

My wife worked part-time in the church office as the pastor's assistant. On Friday, while at work, a co-worker answered the phone. On the line was a man who had no connection to our church. This man said that he had made one phone call to his own church, a group of about 300, found there was no need for his offer, so he continued, "I thought of Christ Community second. I'm calling to see if there is anyone in your church who is 'just starting' a contracting business." The lady on the phone answered that yes, indeed, there was someone. She told of how I had just got my license the previous day. "Well," he continued, "I want to give him my truck. It is a ¾ ton pick-up with ladder rack and tool boxes. Would this new contractor want it?"

When my cell phone rang, three people on the other end—all competing to blurt out the good news—hastily told of this latest development. By late afternoon, I was the new owner of a Ford F350. I remember making the drive to where I would meet the man. Over and over I repeated, "I just can't believe it!" I called my parents in Maine to tell them the story and they, too, were amazed at God's goodness. What I could not know was that it was only just the beginning of the amazing story that was being written. When I picked up the vehicle, the owner said it had a few problems that should be taken care of right away. One was that it needed a brake job. As we signed the necessary documents, he filled me in on the quirks that the truck had . . . and I was on my way.

You might guess that at this point in the story, money was pretty tight. I had not worked in five weeks and paychecks had been bouncing so we had to try to cover all the expenses of bank fees, etc. So now I had a free truck that would need to be parked until enough money could be scraped together to fix it.

I had not driven ten miles from where I received the truck when my cell phone rang. "Scott—hi, it's Doug." Doug was the go-to guy for fixing anything automotive. He owns a small repair shop just outside town. "Scott, why not bring the truck by—I can look it over for you," he continued. I started to protest that I couldn't because we did not have the money to fix it anyway. He pressed a little harder, so I changed course and headed toward Doug. Upon my arrival, he greeted me outside and took a quick glance at the truck. "Leave it here and I will have it repaired within a day or so,"

Doug offered. What I didn't know: someone had called his shop before I arrived to say that it would be their bill—repairs were paid in full!

I had been going to church my whole life, always had a desire to know God and to live like a "good Christian." Through all the years, I had heard stories about, say, someone who didn't have any food, prayed for God to supply it . . . a knock came at the door . . . and someone stood there with a bag of groceries. But that was someone else . . . not me. I never expected anything like that—*hoped* for, but never expected. Besides, I wasn't even asking for any of this. I never asked for a truck and now, for the truck to be fixed—at no cost to me.

I have been playing with comparisons back and forth between my own story and the story of people from centuries long past. Do I think I am Moses – Abraham – Noah? Definitely not. Do I think that they were men who got up every morning and had to put their sandals on, just like me? Definitely, yes. What I mean to say, these men, whom we regard with reverence— as well we should—did not know anything beyond the minute they lived in. They could only look over their shoulders and review the path they had walked up till this point. They could point to the various incidents where God had met them and take faith that the same God was still at work in their ongoing journey. That is why I am recording my story: their stories give me hope; perhaps mine can offer the same.

I am stunned at how God has been so incredibly faithful to me. Scott, a nobody, a boy from the rolling hills of wooded northern Maine. Why would He even notice me? Well, that causes me to think of the characters I have written about. Why would God notice *anyone*? Abraham is a liar: he said to the king, no, this isn't my wife . . . she's just my sister. Noah—another outstanding example—gets so drunk one night his kids have to drag him into his tent and cover up his naked butt. Why? Why would God choose any of us? Because He is God . . . and He is good! If anyone has the simple trust, like these men, the reward is beyond any amount of descriptive words I can think up. He is at work in all of our lives—all the time. Some respond to that calling and turn to Him and experience life, scripture puts it, life to the full. It is not life without struggle or pain, as you will read in the pages ahead, but it is life, and . . . He is good.

So far, we are only at the point of Friday afternoon. Wednesday I took the test, Thursday the call came that I had passed, now it is Friday and I have picked up my new truck . . . all repairs paid for. Not bad. It gets better. The church we attended was a community of around 120 people. I had been an up-front person every week, leading the band in worship and also one of four elders who governed the church. Almost everyone attending had heard snippets of the story so our pastor took a portion of the worship service to show pictures of the truck on the jumbo screens and allowed me to give details of how the week had played out. Everyone was excited for our family and thanked God for being so generous.

The service ended and several came wishing me well on my new venture. One of the well-wishers, whom I barely knew at the time, asked if our family needed meat. I have always found it hard to accept anything. Somewhere in me is this idea that you should earn what you get. So I told him we were doing okay. Small untruth—I had not received a paycheck in over a month and we had four children to feed. He insisted that I come by his shop the next day. What I didn't know was that he owned a butcher shop. By the next evening we had enough meat to nearly fill a chest freezer. I could not believe it! I was unemployed, no paycheck . . . but enough Porterhouse steaks to give away. The writer of Matthew records Jesus saying to live generously as He has lived towards us. I felt like opening our front door and inviting the city over for a giant block party—I'll bring the meat.

At some point, during this whirlwind of activity since the Sunday night of deciding to start a business, I had sat down and made up a wish list of tools I would like to purchase.

I had taken time to research where I could get them and who had the best price. Another man greeted me on that Sunday morning. Again, it was someone I did not know very well. His question was whether I need any tools. I told him I had quite a few but could always use more, half in a joking manner. I never thought any more of it until the doorbell woke me from my traditional Sunday afternoon nap.

Now—standing in front of me—was the man who had inquired if I needed any tools only hours before. He held out a brand new saw. Not just any saw—the exact expensive one that I wanted. What do you do?! I just stood there with the door open in disbelief. This can't be true! His wife, whom I knew only a fraction better than her husband, reported to me later that she, too, was shocked. Her husband wasn't like that, she said. He wouldn't even do that for himself—never mind doing it for someone he barely knew.

Time after time during that season God kept pouring out His provision on us. Another story: our family was on the way to help a good friend move her office. While we were stopped at a red light, I noticed a friend behind us. She was a very outgoing person, so it didn't seem too strange that she would get out of her car and come up to my door. Thinking she was just saying hi, I rolled my window down only to have her tuck something into my shirt pocket and run back to her van. As I took it from my pocket I saw that it was a gas card, when I looked at the gas gauge it was on . . . E.

Why?

Why us?

Were we special?

Did God love us more?

No . . . a million times: No!

25

CHAPTER 5

Consider God

My thoughts are being informed by stories from Scripture. In the Bible there is a book called Hebrews that has a chapter devoted to telling a few stories of men and women who dared to believe what God said. It is called: *faith*. They had no reason to believe anything other than they felt like it was God telling them to act on what they had heard. I have already written about how ridiculous some of the things were that these men and women believed. Yet, there is a chapter devoted to them, to which many refer as the "Faith Hall of Fame." On one hand, I do not consider myself to be among those who stand on that stage of heavyweights. Yet, in another sense, anyone who has ever had courage to act on words that God has given is absolutely qualified to stand shoulder to shoulder with them. You may never be asked to build a supersized boat and call animals two by two; never be told that a great nation will come from your offspring; never be . . . *fill in the blank*. But you are called: called to believe that God is, and that He is calling people to trust Him. Trust that He absolutely knows the best way to live life. If we follow that, it will be good. In our culture, that may appear to be just as ridiculous as any one of the stories I have already mentioned. We are sophisticated . . . enlightened . . . too grown up to believe in an unseen God who wants to be involved in our story. Whether we like it or not—believe in God, or not—He is in control. He continues to want to go back to the story from the very beginning of time. Genesis says that God walked in the garden with Adam and Eve. That is what He wants to do again. He wants to walk with us and tell us of His incredible plan for our lives.

All of that is to say, I am no better or worse than the rest of humanity. The distinction is that I dared to believe what God was saying for my life. My response felt like a T.V. commercial from my childhood: where a relaxed, fully trusting, no-worries-in-the-world person . . . fell backwards into a pristine pool of water in a move that came to be known as the "Nestea Plunge." I have tried to re-enact that. It is almost impossible to do. I always look over my shoulder to be sure the pool of water that I am about to fall into has not mysteriously emptied in the last two seconds. I want to know there is something there to soften my fall. Like in a favorite *Indiana Jones* scene: Harrison Ford needs to cross a huge canyon, he can't see anything, yet the legend says that when he makes one step there will be a bridge under his feet. There are times when that is exactly what it feels like. We are asked to trust so completely in something that is absolutely crazy. What I have found to be true is that when you do, the reward is beyond anything that can be imagined. There is, indeed, water in the pool. Why didn't I see that bridge there all the time?

Paul, a man who wrote the majority of the New Testament, tells the church in Rome that a Godly life is "life filled with expectancy." There are times when I think the church has lost that sense of wonder. It has become dry and some may even say boring and irrelevant to our modern lifestyle. Being a Christian was never meant to be a dull list of rules to follow just to avoid being incinerated by hell's flames. God's longing is to continually be showing us who He is and how amazing He can be—if we believe what He says.

My path was that He asked me to step outside of the security of doing what I had always done. I have no idea what God is asking you to do. This I do know, though: it will be good. That is not to say that you will get free trucks or gas cards or that your freezer will be filled with meat. It does say that you will be alive—alive in the best sense. Not the mundane existences of working—so you can eat, work, eat, sleep, retire for a few years . . . then die. This life we are given is an amazing gift that calls to us to live it following the God who passionately loves us.

As you read on I will tell how my journey had a very hard passage that almost took my life. Even though I say that, I want you to know something before you read one more paragraph. *God is good! God is with me!* I would never wish anyone to pass through the same grief that was mine . . . but in the same breath, I also say that I would not change one minute of it. Why? Because I met God . . . God of whom I had heard hearsay—more like an acquaintance. But now I know Him; know Him like a brother who sits on the hill and shares coffee in the early morning light; know Him like a counselor to whom I run in the moments when the darkness tries to crush life from me like grain under the millstone.

Now I know Him! I say that with a longing that you, too, could be introduced to this God Who is more incredible than any imagination could ever create. The critics may argue that this is my coping mechanism. The thing that life required of me was too hard for reality, so my mind was tricked into believing in an unseen force that Karl Marx called the "opium for the masses." I counter with, "Even the atheist must believe. They must believe that there is no God. Believe that all there is to this life is the cruel realities of today and . . . tomorrow we die into nothingness." With every fiber that is in me I resist that. I walk along the great lake and look at its beauty or awake to a bird singing outside in the early morning. I hear a lecture of someone who has studied the intricate details of our solar system. It is all too grand and full of order not to have God at the very center of it. If there is any persuasion in my words, I hope for you to consider. Consider God . . . not religion . . . God! Consider that the Book is true; consider that the words, "God so loved that He gave," are *true*—and are for *you* . . . today.

As I mentioned, the road was about to take a curve I never saw coming. If I were the author of my days on this earth, I would not have written the story the way it has gone. I'm not the author—God is! Even though life goes places that hurt and grief is worn like a soggy wool blanket . . . God is good!

I have a confession to make at this point in the story. Up until now I thought it was about me. I thought the spectacular roots of my new company called Community Electric were going to lead to wealth and ease. I envisioned having a crew who did the work while I bid jobs and maintained the office. My years of working with tools were about over—according to my plan. I have always enjoyed travel, so in the back of my mind I thought Community Electric was going to be a vehicle to generate enough wealth to achieve that goal. I could not have been more wrong!

There is no way I can point an accusing finger at Abraham for misunderstanding what God said. God said he was going to have a son by his wife, Sarah. As time went by and there was no son, he began to wonder if he had heard right. The story goes that his wife gave him her servant lady called Hagar, who got pregnant and had a child. He must have been thinking he was helping God out. That was not what God intended. He said what He meant: his *wife* was going to have a son. Well . . . I, too, missed the mark on God's plan for my having a business. As it turned out, Community Electric was not so much for generating income; instead, it gave me the ability to be close to my family as dark days loomed on the horizon.

As you have read the account, you might be inclined to say that God was absolutely involved in the lives of Scott and Annette Roix. Life had begun to fall into place. After coming through the unnerving season of being unemployed to the stunning beginning of a new company, we felt as though we were headed back towards the top of the mountain. Business contracts began to fall into place: a good friend, who happened to be a CPA, came over for dinner to offer his services to do the business books for the fledgling company for a year . . . *for free*. Things were coming together. Obviously, this was the place I was meant to be. What I could not know was that I was about to experience God, as I never had before. Every song I had ever sung . . . every sermon I'd ever heard—all were building blocks of a foundation of faith in my life. My footings were about to be tested. There were going to be moments in the months to come when I would feel that the whole thing would come crashing to the ground . . . all that would remain would be a heap of ash.

I have no idea who you are or where you might be on the path of living a life of faith in God. I write with a desire to have a conversation with all who might pick up this book. I wish you could feel how tangible both faith—*and* doubt—were, inside of me. I so wanted to believe that God was with us . . . but, in the same moment, wondered if there even was a God. I wanted to believe "words" that people would say—there were many; I will explain more about that later. I kept asking God if the Bible was true. You may think this is odd. After all, why wouldn't I believe in Him? I had just gotten a free truck.

My mind again turns to Moses. I left off where this once-prince of Egypt—now shepherd in the desert—is listening to a bush. God gives him instruction on what to say to Pharaoh when he approaches the throne. That seems a little thin for the sheep herder. He tells God something to the effect of, "Like, he is going to *believe* that!" God says, "No really . . . I will be with you!" Moses resists again, asking for something a little more solid. "Ok," God says, "what is in your hand?" Moses responds that he is carrying a simple shepherd's staff. "Well . . . throw it on the ground." Moses obeys, and the stick becomes a snake. You might think that he heads back to the farm to drop off the lambs so he can immediately head for Pharaoh's palace. Nope . . . he said something like, "Uhhh . . . God? Could you give me another sign? That one was good and all, but I'm still not sure it's You." God gives him a horrible skin disease one minute, then as quickly as it came, God made it vanish. Now we, as the reader in the 21st century, are thinking, *This guy has got to be on his way. The only thing left is for God to step onto the desert floor and draw him a picture.* Nope . . . not moving. The next line in the story, Exodus 4:13, has Moses telling God, *"O Lord, please send someone else to do it."* Are you kidding me?! Is he dumb as a rock or what? God does all of that to prove He is with this desert dweller and he can't believe it. *I'm no better.*

There are markers all over my path pointing toward God's being with me. So now who is dumb for questioning? I felt like Moses asking, *Please . . . could You just give me one more sign that You are with me before I go?*

I mentioned earlier, *words* from God. I believe God still speaks to His creation by various means, one being what many in Christian circles call "prophetic words." I'm not going to go into a long explanation here as to why I believe that, but my scriptural understanding leads me to believe it. During this time, there were many of those . . . *words* . . . occurring around our life. At the beginning of this season a card came in the mail. A very good friend had written that she had been praying for our family and kept coming back to the same word: transition. She told us that she offered no explanation other than she felt as though God wanted us to know something was in transition in our lives. We had no idea what to make of it, but felt it important to keep in front of our thoughts, so we placed her card beside the kitchen sink and often reread her words. The next significant *word* came a short time later. A college friend who pastors on the east coast called one evening. He and I have a great relationship but talk infrequently—with anywhere from six to ten weeks between conversations. I was eager to fill him in on the recent events. I recall his saying that he had been praying for me and God wanted him to let me know: "I have passed the test and been found not wanting." Again, he offered no explanation other than his sense was that God wanted me to know that. My friend could not have known how important those words were to become. He was willing to go out on a limb and let me know what he sensed God was saying.

Storm clouds had already begun to form over our life. Had it not been for these two friends in particular, along with many more to follow, I think I would have been destroyed. I'll explain in more detail later . . . I do not mean only metaphorically. I write this to let you know how powerful words are. Scripture says that they have the power of life . . . and death. I know it is true. Jesus said, Matthew 4:4, that we need more than bread to stay alive—we need *"a steady stream of words from God's mouth."* Throughout the next months . . . that is exactly what I received.

CHAPTER 6

Dance Partners

Thanksgiving Day, 2007. Our family joined the larger family of brothers and sisters, nieces and nephews, to celebrate and gorge on too much food. We traveled the forty-five minutes to, as I call her, "Momma Margaret's." For some time, leading up to this day, Annette had been experiencing what she thought was pre-menopause symptoms even though it seemed a bit premature. Although she was concerned and had gone for checkups, it seemed that overall she was doing okay. Doctors did not have reason to be alarmed. Unknown to me, on that day of giving thanks, our family's whole world was about to change.

As the family was going about the business of preparing the large feast, Nette was hemorrhaging in the bathroom—copious amounts of blood! At this point, she did not want to draw attention to herself, so she quietly pulled her mom aside after lunch. As they began doing Internet research, it appeared that there could be any number of reasons for what she had experienced: one of them, cancer.

Of course it's not *that*! Annette was thirty-eight and in great shape. Besides being an active mom, she also regularly worked out at the YMCA. There was no reason to think that this was anything beyond a bad urinary tract infection. The first I heard of it was during the ride home. Annette reported that she would like to drop the kids and me off and then go to the emergency room . . . *alone.*

This word "alone" was to come up a lot over the next months. Annette was on a quest to find out who she was. The question that persisted in her thoughts at the time was who *was* she apart from her role as wife and mother? She had only months earlier taken the youth on a mission trip to Mexico, and upon her return seemed to be a completely changed person—a person I did not know. The way she responded to me changed; there was an edge now, a coldness that I was not used to after sixteen years of marriage. Something had shifted and I did not see it coming.

Annette meant so much to me. I did not understand what was happening. I became very disoriented. Why wouldn't my wife want me to go to the E.R. with her?

The doctor on duty that night did the exam and prescribed meds to treat a urinary tract infection, but thought it was important that she be checked by our family physician as soon as possible. That man was Dr. Jeff Capes. What an incredible gift he became to our family. He was a well-trained professional and a caring human being. For both those things we were thankful. Dr. Capes saw Nette and ordered a battery of tests trying to find the source of bleeding. As Nette was about to head off to complete the battery of tests that had been ordered, her cell rang. Dr. Capes said, "Hi, Nette. I was thinking about you and there is one more test that I think we should do." It wasn't until later that Dr. Capes reported that it was that particular test that showed him what he did not want to see. It was a Wednesday afternoon, around suppertime, on a cold, dark, dreary, late fall day—a day I will never forget. The phone rang. It was one of those calls that you can't wait to answer and yet dread beyond words at the same time. Annette took the call, next thing I knew, she was slumped into her chair . . . handing the phone to me. "Hi Scott, Jeff Capes calling." The words that followed all began to slur together. Words that were to become part of our routine vocabulary . . . at this point were alien: renal cell carcinoma. I have heard others who experience trauma report that time and space seems to slow to a frame-by-frame . . . every second as long as a minute. I remember where I was standing . . . how the furniture was arranged . . . who was there—I see it all. "Scott, we want to schedule Annette for surgery as soon as possible." From the test that had been run, Dr. Capes determined that there was a large mass growing in the kidney. The next two weeks were a blur of activity. Schedules reworked. Things that at one time—only moments before—were huge . . . now diverted by a new urgency: surgery.

At the time I began Community Electric, I had wrestled with the thought of whether I should stay union or not. For a small contractor it was very expensive. The monthly dues and insurance were heavy. I soon appreciated the choice to stay. Medical bills, coming almost daily, soon approached $700,000. One bill in particular came from the pharmacy for $170,000. God had guided our steps, like He promised He would. Because of the excellent benefits, we were able to seek the best medical treatment available. The kidney was removed . . . and prognosis looked good.

Soon after surgery, Nette had an appointment with an oncologist. After reviewing lab tests on the dissected organ, it was almost certain that the surgeon had got all of it. From all appearances, this episode seemed to be a shot across the bow letting us know . . . life is a gift. Even as I say that it sounds like such a bumper sticker. I'm not sure anyone who has not faced the prospect of death can fully appreciate how true the words are.

In the telling of my story I want to convey more than dates, times and events. I want it to be a glimpse inside of my walk with God. I have made comparisons of the lives of heroes of Scripture with my own. The last time I spoke of Moses he was reluctantly headed towards Pharaoh's office for an audacious request. God had said to go tell the most powerful ruler in the world to release the vast majority of his workforce . . . so they could go worship. To me, that seems like the most ridiculous thing in the world! Something similar to that would be knocking on the White House door demanding our troops come home—immediately. Probably wouldn't make much headway. Moses did it though. I picture him approaching the steps that lead up to Pharaoh's high throne. He climbs one . . . two—doubt mounting with every movement forward. He may even have reversed his steps. *No way! This is insane! God didn't say that.* Ultimately, we know that Moses did do it.

I also imagine that after each time God did what He said He could and would do, Moses became a little bolder in doing what God asked. In my life I, too, have carried the uncertainty of knowing if God really, really, *really* said it . . . or was it just my own wishful thinking?

Tension between dance partners—faith and doubt—is nothing new. John the Baptist, the man who heralded with such certainty when he saw Jesus coming to be baptized, "Here he is . . . this is the man I have been talking about," in a few more chapters, now sits in prison asking a few of his friends to "go ask if He really is the one . . . or should we keep looking for another?" Why is it that when life throws a curve we doubt God? Is He only God when all is good? I say to myself that my faith is not that shallow, yet I lay awake at night wondering about next steps. Did I really understand what God said? From the core of who I am I want to know God, want to know if He can still do those "ridiculous" things He used to do in centuries past. Maybe . . . perhaps . . . could it be that living a life of faith is not boring? It is more than a duty of going to church to assuage our conscience? There is so much more we can see if only we had a little bit of faith—even just a seed.

In moments when I think the life I am walking is madness, I take hope in reading the accounts from the bestselling book in the world—the Bible. I think of the amazing reward of living a life following after God. Moses could have stayed a shepherd in the desert until his dying day. He would have missed out on really living. This simple shepherd would never have seen all the incredible signs that God did before Pharaoh would send the slave nation on their way. His eyes would never have witnessed the sea opening to allow people to cross to the other side. This simple desert dweller was able to see God . . . all because he chose to trust.

In me is such a hunger to experience more from life, even when it is hard. As long as God is with us, it will be okay. Moses came to the place in his journey of faith where it is recorded in Exodus 33:15 that he said, "I will not go . . . if you (God) do not go with me." The days I have been telling of were extremely hard; they were the hardest I had ever lived through. Yet, I *knew* that God, the One Who kept drawing me towards this life of belief, was with me.

Nette continued to recover from surgery. The oncologist report was good; however, she was asked to consider being a part of a clinical study—sort of insurance in case there were any remaining cells. The days leading up to the trial were agonizing. Should she endure the uncomfortable side effects for a year and a half . . . or chance that there were no remaining cancer cells roaming free in her body? Ultimately, the thought that if she did nothing and cancer returned was too much. She began the first round of experimental medicine two months following surgery.

I need to give you a glimpse into the relationship piece as well as the physical. After recovering from the removal of the kidney, Nette began to revisit the places in her mind pre-cancer. Only now they became magnified. Here is what I mean. Annette had joined a cancer support group that also offered gifted counselors to help navigate this new reality. The counselor said that often a traumatic event, such as cancer at 38, could trigger a mid-life crisis. For us, it did! Nette set out to prove she was a strong woman; she could do it alone. She did not need me; did not want me. The rejection was almost intolerable. I was consumed with my wife; the thought of losing her was unbearable. I lay on my bed and shivered as if a window had been left open on a winter night . . . but it was not *that kind* of cold. It was the all-consuming thoughts of my wife leaving me. My emotions vacillated: loving her more than anything, yet so angry at her selfishness towards the kids and me. My confusion came from not knowing how my wife could lean on me for everything over the last several months only to come to the place where she would say, "I don't want you to say 'I love you' anymore."

This writing is about our story; it is bigger than that, though. It is about God and His activity in our lives. This is why I tell how dark it was: so that later it will show how brilliant the light of God is. I am quite sure that if it were not for Christ's example of showing how to love, my future would have looked very different. In no way do I mean to smear the name of my wife. I only offer details that Annette and I shared publicly. My motive is to offer hope to anyone who may read these words and identify with my feelings of despair. Prior to living through this experience I would have said something to the effect, "How could life be so bad that anyone would want to kill himself?" I was experiencing how bad!

On one of my return trips from a jobsite, the tormenting thoughts of "what if?" kept rolling over and over. It felt like someone continually hitting the replay button without mercy. As I drove, the thought crossed my mind of what would happen if I were to veer off the road aimed towards the concrete bridge abutment. It would appear like an accident so the kids could have the insurance money, and I could escape the pain of life. Today, I am thankful that I did not have the courage to act on my thoughts. I wasn't thankful that day! After completing a sixty-plus mile commute, I arrived home. Just as I was backing my truck into the driveway, a weld broke. The passenger side tire broke free and went completely to the front of the wheel well—there was no way to control the truck. I was so mad! Why couldn't that have happened on the interstate while doing seventy-five miles an hour? No . . . no, that would have been too easy. When the tow truck came to pick up the vehicle, I ran the scenario by the driver. "What would have happened if this would have let go while driving down the road?" His response to me was "Buddy, you would have been end over end in the ditch. You could not have controlled that truck." It seemed to me God had more for me—my time was not complete.

CHAPTER 7

It Is for Purpose

Annette and I agreed that something needed to change. Travel arrangements were made for Nette to have a two-week getaway for her to sort through her thoughts. There would be no communication once she got to her destination—I emphasize how odd that was: we talked about everything. Now . . . silence. Disoriented, confused, angry. Pride—some may say arrogance. I thought our marriage was different than this. After all, we were "Christians." This couldn't happen to *us*. Yet, here we were, and I felt powerless to change anything. It seemed like the hand was being played out and all I could do was to lay down the cards that were dealt to me.

Again, I refer to quote/unquote, "word of the Lord." There were hundreds of people praying for us. Since December, when cancer was first discovered, Nette had been recording her thoughts on a blog that soon developed a large following across the globe. Some who had been praying felt like God was speaking to them, either through a thought or a verse from Scripture. Many would call or write to say what they felt God might want to communicate with us, the Roix family. I remember how much strength I felt from these words. One that repeated itself seven times by seven different people from different regions of the United States said that what we were living through "was for purpose". I held onto those words as tightly as someone who has capsized hangs onto a life ring. They were my hope.

I could not imagine what sort of purpose a 38-year-old wife and mother having cancer could serve. What purpose is there for a troubled relationship that by all appearances looked to be headed to the statistical heap of failed marriages? I believed God. It was all I had. The characters I have written about . . . it was all they had—a word, a thought, a verse. They acted on their belief . . . and God was with them. It was faith. I think I am forever changed from living any other way. He has done the most amazing things in my life . . . taken me places I could only dream of and some I never could have. So I trust. Trust that whatever purpose there is, He knows and sees and most importantly . . . walks with.

Nette was seven days into her solitude when she phoned to ask if I would join her for the second half. She said there were things that we needed to talk about. It felt like déjà vu of the night she returned from the women's conference. I was a little skeptical, to be sure. My answer was not an automatic yes. First, I phoned two close friends who had been aware of our situation, seeking their advice. Both gave an enthusiastic *yes.* Travel plans were made to join Nette on Wednesday and we both would return on Saturday.

Just hours before I was to board the plane to go to where my wife was waiting, the plan was interrupted. Now, I was headed to a new destination—one that would impact the rest of my life. I have an aversion to using clichés or religious sayings—they turn my stomach. When I say it felt like we were *carried* through the next several days, I pour every ounce of meaning that can be given to the word *carried.* I do not mean some religious lingo—I *know* Christ was the guide who helped us navigate the most dangerous waters we had ever been through. I offer no details other than on the first day of coming together, our conversation lasted more than ten hours. From there we were able to make forward progress with the aid of gifted counselors that met with us three times a week.

The Bible refers to one called Satan. It says that this power of darkness comes only to kill, steal, and destroy what is good. The plan for complete destruction of our family was evident. The story could have looked so different had it not been for humility and courage to trust and believe the best.

Again, "the word of the Lord" came to us on the last day as we packed our bags to return home. This time it was a family member who called to say that as they were driving they felt like God was telling them things to share with us. It became so urgent that they pulled the vehicle to the side of the road and began to capture the thoughts on paper—words that would both comfort and instruct for the days ahead. I carry a copy in my computer bag and often reference that which gave so much hope. There was no way this family member had any understanding of the meaning of what they were sharing; to me, it felt like a giant overhead spotlight illuminating the darkness. God knew where we were; not only knew, but also cared—enough to communicate things to my heart that only I knew. Here are a few of the lines: "I was shaping you with experience, there was no other way. I have hundreds of children, even thousands, that don't understand my love—how deep, how real, how life changing it really is. I knew you would not be able to minister without experience. I knew you could not understand unless you had been there in the darkness." There is a song our congregation would often sing, "I am a Friend of God." A line from one of the stanzas asks, "Who am I, that you are mindful of me?" Those words became even more meaningful to me God of all creation . . . God Who speaks and things come into being . . . God—*He* is aware and mindful of our plight while we journey. It seems too grand to comprehend, but it is not my idea to be a friend of God's, it was His! He (God) showed that to all humanity by joining us on this sphere called earth. Christ absolutely showed us how to live life. He did not come pointing a scolding finger accompanied with words of shame and "You ought to . . ." Instead, He came and lived it before us; showed us how to respond when the one we love *rejects* us. Peter, one of Christ's closest companions, one who shared some of the most incredible moments like walking on water and witnessing jaw-dropping miracles; when pressed by onlookers, said, "No . . . no, I don't know that #+$%&-@* man." This once intimately close student then turned and ran as if he had never crossed paths with the man called Christ. I often wonder if Jesus heard that denial from his closest friend. Did those words cut deeper than the whips from the Roman guards? Jesus then did the most unusual—unnatural—thing. The next time Jesus saw Peter, the first words exchanged were: *Peace.* As if to say, "It's o.k. Peter, I forgive you." Here is a dilemma: if I am indeed a follower of Christ and that is how He handled rejection . . . it seems there isn't any question of what I should do. Otherwise, why pretend? Why follow any of the teaching from the Jewish rabbi? He was not offering *suggestions* on how to live. He said follow Me; do what I do—it leads to life.

Annette and I were committed to God and each other. The days were not easy, but as we were to soon find out, they were days that also brought healing. Once again we found ourselves on ground that was quite unfamiliar. New fledgling company, kidney cancer, upheaval in a sixteen-year marriage—all within the same year! Emotions ran from despair to exhilaration. In so many ways I felt alive, free from the mundane of everyday life. God accomplished things that leave me amazed to this day.

Annette and I were riding home on a Saturday night during the time we were rebuilding our relationship. I remember just expressing a wish to her. "Nette," I said, "I wish we could find a cabin to go to." My thought was that it would be less confining than a hotel room; we could each have space to ourselves for a while then be together when we desired. That's all I said . . ."I wish." The next morning at church a lady came to Nette and said that she had been praying for us and wondered if we would like to use her fully stocked condo in Door County, Wisconsin. I don't think I am reading too much into it when I say that God was granting even our wishes. We accepted the offer and enjoyed a four-night retreat. It was the calm before the next enormous storm that lurked on our horizon.

CHAPTER 8

Entering the Unknown

In case you lost your way along the timeline, here is a condensed version: kidney removed in December, clinical trial began in February at about the same time our relationship crisis came to a boil and Nette goes on a personal retreat, a month of intense counseling, then the weekend in Wisconsin. Phew—can I finally catch my breath? Not quite! We returned from Door County on Monday afternoon. The following day was the first scheduled C.T. scan since beginning the experimental meds. For the most part, Annette was feeling great. The side effects to the meds were bearable and she was regaining energy that she had not had in several months. Each morning we started the day with a workout at the YMCA or a run through the streets of Ottawa. The C.T. was routine; nothing to worry about. However, cancer, once diagnosed—the word crouches in the shadows of the mind. Nette often said she no longer felt "safe" in her body. It had failed once, so it was not a question of *if*, but *when* it would fail again.

It was a Saturday morning when the call came saying the results were ready to be picked up at the lab. I was enjoying the early June day riding my motorcycle when Nette called to ask if I would stop at the hospital to pick up the results. Neither of us was prepared for the words: suspicious of metastasis—both lungs. Boom. Another blow that dropped us to our knees. The words were right there in black and white. I saw them, understood their meaning—yet could not comprehend. We tried hard not to fall over the edge of the huge cavernous pit of despair. Perhaps we weren't reading the results right? It only says suspicious . . . maybe it isn't anything. We found it difficult not to be anxious until we heard the doctor's interpretation.

The following week, we sat before the oncologist at the local hospital. His grim expression spoke louder than the words he carefully chose. He offered the opinion that if it were his wife he would get to a large medical center that was on the cutting edge of research. I recall leaving his office. I had to will my legs to carry me to the car, my mind a locomotive filled with thoughts that were already a long way down the track. Fear gripped icy fingers around me; it was a death sentence! Doctors had told us from the beginning the cure for kidney cancer was removal of the kidney. Now that it had escaped, primary targets were lungs . . . bone . . . and brain. It had attacked both lungs in six short months.

Life was again taking us places we never had expected to go. I was exhausted! My emotions felt as if they were strapped into the most brutal Six Flags amusement ride. I had just begun to catch my breath from the last traumatic event. Now—here we were faced with the very real prospect of death within six to eight months. My faith began to waiver. Could God do anything? Our young daughter asked, "If God can heal Mom . . . why wouldn't He?" I had no good answer. I suppose I could have given the right "theological" answers that people were offering to us—they seemed so hollow, though. Was God good? Now I was no longer a bystander *watching* the great tragedy of life . . . our family was *in* the drama.

The simple fixes from well-meaning, "loving" people turned my stomach. "Well, you know if you were the head of your house, Scott, then this cancer could not stay," was one bit of advice I got. "Perhaps if you said prayers in a certain way . . ." "Recited certain scriptures . . ." then God would answer. It was overwhelming. These well-meaning Christians felt superstitious: if I massaged Bible verses like some sort of rabbit's foot, then God would hear. Many times their words felt abusive.

Job writes about his good intentioned friends that sat with him when he walked through his nightmare . . . Something about suffering makes observers uncomfortable. Job's company found it difficult to just be with Job. They had to say something; had to make sense of the nonsense. There had to be a reason for the place of misery in which their friend found himself. Surely he had sinned, they assumed; what other explanation could there be? They were wrong. Absolutely wrong. They did not see the larger picture of what was taking place. God was involved, to be sure; He was doing something completely separate from what anyone believed was happening.

The transformation in me has been *to just trust.* Trust . . . no matter the outcome—good or bad—just *trust.* None of us have the luxury, or the burden for that matter, of knowing the end from the beginning. That is reserved for God . . . and God alone. He has the complete panoramic view of life. If I can trust that He sees and knows all things, then why can't I trust Him to be with me through the difficult places?

I will not lie and say that it came without a fight. Of course I fought. "God, what are you doing?" "Why are you taking the one I love?" Prayers vacillated from hope . . . to despair . . . to frustrated anger—all shaken together like a well-stirred cocktail. The way I found rest for my warring mind was in realizing that I am not in control. I cannot figure out the right combination of words to say, prayers to pray, or scriptures to read. God is God. That is it! I . . . along with hundreds of others around the world made it known to God: "Please do not take Nette." I assume somewhere in that mixture of prayers that at least *one* was prayed with faith that He could—and would—heal.

What happens to our belief system when the big Magician in the sky doesn't respond the way we want? What then? Well, He is either not good or not real at all. There is at least one more answer. I think it is the choice that Job had before him. Do as his wife suggested, "Curse God and die; this is all there is to life: pain . . . misery . . . then death, so just get on with it—curse." Believe me, the thought crossed my mind. I had some pretty intense words for God as I drove down the highway—in my *free* truck. Oh, the irony of it. I could believe God gave me the truck. Who could dispute that? Yet I railed against Him in the pain of the present. What?! Is He the cosmic candy man or what? I came across the meaning of Israel the other day: "God wrestler." That is exactly what I was doing. Wrestling with all that I thought I knew. Wrestling with what people were telling me about Him. Who are you God; what do you want? Job did not take his wife's suggestion. Instead, he decided to trust. He did not do it perfectly. The end of the story is God calling for Job to step outside his tent. "Hey, Job, come out here—I got a few questions for you. You think you're so smart? Well, answer these questions . . ." I won't take the time to write all of the questions that God posed to Job—I urge you to read Job, chapter 38, in the *Message* Bible.

The inquiries of God show how absolutely grand He is. Vocabulary escapes human mouths when trying to describe God. His plans and purposes are incredibly higher than my mind can comprehend. With my limited perspective, how could I know what "purpose" this could serve? Slowly, my prayers began to shift—less wrestling, more listening.

Christ's prayer only hours before He was to be impaled to a tree had two parts. He told God what he wanted: "Please, Father, let this pass from me." *I paraphrase: "Please come up with another plan besides this."* His prayer does not stop there, though, with only the request to remove pain. Again, I paraphrase: *"You know what I want, but You know what is best. You know the end before it starts.*" He didn't say it, but it is definitely implied—I trust You!

I have found the most incredible freedom in those words. Whatever my life is—good or bad—He knows what is going on. One day, perhaps I will understand better.

Once again, the transition was made from the shock and anguish of the current diagnosis to putting on the game face— how can this be beat? Annette was in great physical shape. She looked and felt the best she had in years. By every indication, she was the best (if there is such a thing) type of candidate to fight this disease.

Because of the excellent health insurance provided through the electrical union, we were able to seek the best medical care available. We found that in Dr. Regina Stein, an oncologist from Northwestern Memorial Hospital in downtown Chicago. She is an amazing person with whom we had the privilege to cross paths. Our first introduction to Dr. Stein came in December when the option of being a part of the clinical trial was offered. Now, following the advice of local physicians, we once again sought her expertise. Like Dr. Capes, Dr. Stein became a lot more to us than an aloof medical professional. From the very first encounter she made it very clear that she intended to fight this intruder to the very end . . . and that she did. She later told me at a lunch appointment that when she looked at the client list for the day and saw Annette Roix's name, she had a sinking feeling.

In December, everything had looked so clean—promising. Now, only six months later, it had progressed to numerous locations—in both lungs. Immediately, Dr. Stein put together a plan to attack the intruding cells. She explained it would be the most aggressive meds that could be given called Interleukin II (IL 2). There was almost a 100% guarantee that Annette would be in intensive care within the first day once the medicine was started. Dr. Stein did not try to conceal how difficult these rounds of treatment would be. She did think it had the best chance of beating metastatic cancer. Reminiscent of December, there began a flurry of appointments and testing to assure that Annette's body could indeed take the maximum dose.

Up to this point, the church community we attended had been incredibly generous towards our family; somehow, they found yet another gear. Just days before the intense treatments were to begin, a group of friends gathered as a think-tank to consider how our needs could be met. Charts began forming to cover everything from food to childcare to transportation to cleaning the house to lawn care to pet care . . . everything. We were immersed in loving hands. All our needs were being provided for.

One friend, who had been in a small group with us, parked his brand new Envoy in our driveway. He wanted us to have a comfortable vehicle while driving back and forth to Chicago. Comfortable — I'll say! Leather interior, moon roof, multiple CD changer, power everything, and most important . . . A/C. Our aging van did not have a reliable air conditioner; now, our need was met without even asking. The same friend came to me almost every Sunday and quietly slipped hundred dollar bills into my hand. "Here, Scott—you probably need gas." This is not a wealthy man; he works days . . . nights . . . weekends, just like everybody else. He was teaching me a lesson. The experience was humbling and incredibly thrilling. At the moment of our greatest need in life, the Body of Christ — the church — carried us.

I say it was humbling because I often felt obligated to repay anytime someone offered help. I was powerless; there was no possible way to repay all the generosity we were being shown. Thirty people showed up at the house to clean toilets, trim shrubs, empty and straighten cabinets, wash walls—not once, but multiple times. I do not know how people do life alone; it is something I hope never to experience.

Another friend who attended the initial think-tank session offered his talent to put together a benefit. Even though insurance was now covering 100% of the bills, there were still enormous needs to be met. Back and forth to Chicago, parking, meals, hotel . . . Yeah, you get it; it was not cheap! Our friend assembled a team that worked extremely hard. By the day of the benefit, local shopkeepers had donated hundreds of dollars in merchandise. Late into the night, the phone rang. We were asked to guess how much money had been raised. Annette and I guessed by the size of the crowd it was probably around thirteen thousand dollars. No. No, it was way more than that. In that single event — with matching funds from Lutheran Life — over *forty thousand dollars* had been raised.

Worship the next day felt like static electricity filling the air. What an amazing God!! I know I am repeating myself when I say it was the most difficult time in our life; but in the same breath I add that God was unmistakably involved in all of it. The threat of death caused us to live.

The day of the first round of treatment began with yet another generous gift. A couple, who are more like a brother and sister than friends, arranged for Annette and me to kayak our favorite section of the river. The early morning was absolutely perfect. We glided down the bluff-lined waterway talking of all that God had done in our life together: how we had come together on a small college campus in Dover, Delaware, the high points, and laughing at our children's antics. Anyone observing along the shore could have never guessed the punishing toll meds were about to take on this beautiful kayaker in a few short hours. As we pulled the boats from the water, our friends had chosen a shelter to prepare a breakfast that included champagne goblets for orange juice. Extravagant!

David, another character from Scripture, had a similar experience of generosity. He mused aloud that he would like a drink of water from the well where he had spent his childhood. The trouble was that an enemy army currently occupied it. Without his knowledge three of his companions fought their way across the enemy line and brought a container filled with the well water that David had so longed for. David then did the most strange thing . . . he poured it onto the ground. The thing he had only hours earlier wished he could taste, he poured out. He said the cost for that gift was way too high; he poured it out as an offering to God. I get that. The things people had given to us — every generous act, every thoughtful word — were very, very expensive. If these gifts had been water, I think I, too, would have poured it on the ground. These offerings — all the time, energy, inconveniences — all of it, I would have poured out to God. He is the only one worthy of that kind of generosity, not me.

CHAPTER 9

Round #1

The day the PICC line, a main I.V. sight to be used for the upcoming chemo, was inserted, Annette was also scheduled for a lung biopsy. She was wheeled away and I remained in a waiting area. A little over an hour later a nurse came to say that I could join Nette in her recovery room. Annette was alert and talkative and began to tell how the procedure was performed. It involved a long needle being stuck through her chest into her lung. It was more info than my very active imagination could take. The room began to swirl and beads of sweat broke on my forehead! Next thing I knew, Nette, who was lying on a stretcher, was instructing me to take a seat and put my head between my knees. Nice job, Scott. I was there to offer support and almost needed medical assistance myself.

The hour had arrived for us to make our way to Chicago's Northwestern Memorial Hospital. What lay ahead of Annette was terrifying. The internet is a wonderful, yet horrible tool. Wonderful, because it allows patients to be better educated about the care they are receiving; horrible, because there is so much information that it can feel like the mother load of info has been downloaded into your brain. Then we are left to sort what is true versus what is urban legend. Nette spent hours researching IL 2 and the numerous side affects it caused. It did not bring any comfort knowing that in the early stages of the drug, mortality rate was very high.

However, as time passed, doctors and medical staff began to gain perspective on how powerful the medicine was, and the death rate began to get lower. It was with that dread that we drove to our destination. As the Chicago skyline came into view, the small talk that made up our conversation became less and less. There comes a point when words are no longer necessary . . . everything has already been said. There is no vocabulary left that communicates as much as a gentle squeeze of the hand, a stroke of the hand to the nape of the neck; nothing more is needed, just, "I am with you." Nette had come to the place in her heart that she no longer wanted, or for that matter, needed, to be alone.

We entered Prentice Women's Hospital early afternoon in anticipation of the first of fourteen doses that were to be given over the next five days. Each round took fifteen minutes to drip through the recently inserted PICC line in Annette's arm.

Fear of the unknown was taking its toll. Dr. Stein entered the room and Annette could not hold emotions in check any longer; tears flowed. Dr. Stein immediately shifted roles, and that day, she became Regina. She sat on the edge of the bed and wrapped loving arms around a friend. This beautiful connection blossomed into an incredible relationship. All was forever changed as a result of paths crossing.

The plan was that I would take Nette to Northwestern then leave as the first round got under way. Annette's mom, Momma Margaret, would spend the week at the bedside of her baby girl. I would be home with our children, and then return the next weekend to bring Annette home. Leaving was the hardest thing. Within minutes of the medicine entering Annette's body, she began experiencing "rigors"—an involuntary shaking. Her temperature skyrocketed. It was the most helpless feeling. Lying on the bed was a perfectly healthy-looking, beautiful lady. Only hours earlier she had kayaked a scenic river. Now, she was subjected to drugs that held some promise of wiping out the intruding cancer cells that were growing in her lungs.

The drug lived up to its billing. Within a day Nette was moved into intensive care where they were better equipped to monitor vital signs and had a skilled staff to respond if she were to be in crisis. Margaret was tenacious, remaining at the bedside, offering any support she could to the medical staff. The week passed and again, true to the medicine's reputation, it was a week of hell then, shortly after the last dose, the body quickly recovered normal function. Annette recovered so quickly that Northwestern had to consider a request they had never encountered before . . . she went home from ICU! No one had done that before so the nurses did not know the procedure, since there wasn't one. Patients don't often go straight home from Intensive Care! Finally, late Sunday evening, Dr. Stein gave her approval for the uncommon discharge.

Annette was exhausted but relieved that the first week was behind her. Now it was "wait and see" if the horrible experience yielded any benefit. What elation when the CT scan showed the tumors had indeed been affected. They had shrunk ever so slightly . . . but shrunk! I say elation; the truth of it is Nette received the results with mixed thoughts. She was pleased that they had shrunk, but remained skeptical of the lasting effect.

Along the path we were walking, there were signs indicating God's involvement in every way. As Nette was being readied for one of many tests, the attending nurse began to ask about Nette's sickness and diagnosis. People often had to ask because Nette looked perfectly healthy. Annette explained that her diagnosis was terminal cancer with a range of six to eight months to live. The nurse proceeded to ask if she was afraid to die, and Nette affirmed that indeed, she was. The two of them stepped into the hall outside the examining room. Once there, this random, chance encounter with this particular nurse became clearer in purpose. Her story was that when she was fourteen years old something happened—-I'm not certain what happened—but the result was that she was clinically dead! However, her mother prayed, pleading with God not to take her teenage daughter. The nurse continued, "I saw the most amazingly beautiful things while I was in that place. I want to tell you not to be afraid; once you are there, you do not want to be here."

No matter what you call it, "coincidence" or a "God moment," the effect was comfort. Here Nette was in this large medical facility in the heart of Chicago where people are mostly known by a bar code on a wristband; here, in this place, she felt like God gave her that particular nurse on that particular day so she would hear "Don't be afraid." Once more we were reminded that we were not alone on this journey . . . God was with us.

The days of recovery went by quickly. Nette regained her strength and we soon resumed our exercise regime. At this point the prospect of dying in less than a year was informing us that every single day is important. We did not want to waste any of the time we had . . . be it six months or ten years. We began to live intentionally.

The interval between doses of IL 2 was much shorter than any of us would have liked. Nette was feeling great but looked forward to the next round of meds with total dread. She vividly recalled how miserable the treatment had been and was very reluctant to go through that again. A good friend had given our family a painting that she had created several months earlier titled "I have to!" Those words became one of Nette's mantras. "If I want to continue the path to health, I have to go through this," she often said.

The day came when round two was scheduled to start. Once again we made the hour and a half trek to Chicago—this time the whole trip in silence, knowing what she faced. Upon our arrival at Northwestern Memorial we parked in the garage and made our way to check in at the Feinberg portion of the hospital. After completing the necessary paperwork the receptionist said that we should wait there for a minute until a porter could take Nette to her room in a different building called Prentice Women's. Soon a beautiful African-American lady showed up pushing a wheelchair, greeted us with a warm smile, and offered to wheel Nette to her room. Small pleasantries were exchanged as we made our way to the waiting room. When Nette was wheeled into all too familiar surroundings, she could no longer hold her emotions in check. The lady who had brought us to this point, whom I still only know as Yolanda, noticed tears trickling down forming a drip off the end of Nette's chin. Quietly she stood before the wheelchair and gently rested her chin on top of Nette's head. Ever so softly she whispered over and over, "Oh baby, oh baby." Then as if she had some great inspiration, she stopped and began to speak. "Annette, this is not about you." She then turned and pointed towards me, "This is about him. This is about the book that is in him that will affect thousands."

Wow! That was my initial thought. Where did that come from? Poor Nette had to be thinking, *Thanks a lot, buddy . . . I'm the one going through this mess . . . and it's not even about me!* What we found out later is that Yolanda is a pastor who also works for Northwestern. The words she spoke have been confirmed many, many times by a variety of people. Often, as I tell the stories you have been reading, people respond with, "You need to write a book." That is what I'm doing. It seems a little strange; after all, my training is in electrical work and Biblical studies—not writing books! It is not any more strange than a shepherd leading a slave nation or a hundred year old nomad having children. Where it goes from here is up to God. If indeed it does affect thousands, I am a grateful participant in bringing hope to anyone who is walking through life's biggest challenges.

CHAPTER 10

Dread . . . Round #2

The second round of IL 2 began with the same intensity as the first. A chemo-nurse told us IL 2 is not anywhere near as toxic as some chemo-therapies, but it still causes you to do a double take when the nursing staff puts on a hazmat suit before hanging the bag of medicine from the I.V. pole. The nurse said there are some solutions so strong that if it were to contact skin it would burn a hole through it. Yikes. And that stuff is pumped into people's bodies! What a mind God has given mankind to have the ability to produce such things that bring healing to so many.

Annette had been through round one of immuno-therapy; we thought we had a pretty good idea of how the second round would go. It would be a week of feeling absolutely horrible followed by a quick recovery, then a week or so at home. This pattern was to be repeated over several months until finally the last cancerous cells were wiped out. It was not to be.

As before, I delivered Nette to the hospital and stayed until the first chemo bag began to slowly drip into Nette's body. Momma Margaret took up her post once more beside the bed of her youngest child. I returned home to our children and tried doing the routine tasks of daily living. Impossible! Every thought was consumed with how my other half was doing. I tried to concentrate on the work before me, only to be distracted. My mind was tormented from every angle.

Should I be by Nette's bedside, or is that admitting that she is dying? Others thought it best for me to be at home, working. Let me say there was no shortage of what others thought I should be doing. It was maddening! At times it felt like no matter what I did, it would not be right.

July 31, 2008, two days into round two. Some very good friends took me to supper at a favorite restaurant overlooking the Illinois River. The three of us had just ordered drinks and appetizers when my cell phone rang. "Hi Scott, It's Regina." I knew from the tone of her voice it was not good news. My heart beat faster. I had been updated on developments throughout the day and knew they were having a difficult time regulating blood pressure and heart rate. "Scott, you should return to Chicago." She continued, "We are forced to cease treatments due to a heart arrhythmia that developed." I had a pretty good idea what that meant; still, I asked the question that was at the front of my mind. "How long does she have?" Reminiscent of the December phone call announcing the cancerous kidney, I needed to know the professional opinion, yet did not want to hear the words. This doctor, who had become friend, offered her educated guess that Nette had about nine months to live from the first sign of metastasis— we had already used two! Slowly it began to sink in: I was going to lose my wife in seven months.

Here I stood, in a spot that held incredible memories. Meals shared . . . filling conversations . . . beautiful scenery . . . gentle warm breeze . . . the sounds of summer. It now became the spot of news that was to alter the course of my life's journey. Sobs of grief welled up from the center of my being. Unashamedly, I wept before people who were dining on that beautiful summer evening. I returned to the table where my two friends sat awaiting the news that had obviously shaken me. Once I regained composure I retold the words told to me moments earlier. With a flurry of activity, the bill was paid and I was rushed home to pack a bag and then race for Chicago.

The ride to the city was one of longing . . . and dread. I longed to be at Nette's bedside, to hold her—being true to my words: I will not leave. But there was an overwhelming dread that accompanied the longing. I knew Dr. Stein was withholding the latest development from Nette until my arrival. That Envoy became more than a gift of comfortable transportation from point to point . . . it was a sanctuary! Soft leather embraced my shoulders that were racked with sobs. XM radio playing classical music soothed the ache that was forming in the pit of my soul. The open moon roof allowed the wind to be like the fingers of God tussling my hair. The hour and a half drive was the time I needed to pull myself together enough to stand before my wife as she was told the new development. My premature arrival and ashen look told the story before any words were spoken.

Nette remained in intensive care for another day, and then due to the arrhythmia, was moved to the cardiac floor.

In the story you have been reading I have repeatedly emphasized how much God was involved in every way; still, I vacillated! Hope and despair—sometimes within the same moment. I believed God could do absolutely anything, but *would* He? Since everything was now outside of any control we thought we had, all that was left was to trust God for the unfolding story. We had tried the best medical care we could find; medicine failed. It is really, *really* hard to live with an open hand. A song I often sang had the lines, " . . . the Lord gives . . . the Lord takes away . . . my heart will choose to say, 'Blessed be Your Name!'" The tempo, the range, the whole arrangement of music made it one of my favorite songs to sing. My life of following Christ was now honing in with laser intensity on whether I believed it—or not.

Now what? What should we do? There were several schools of thought; I will boil it down to two. We could follow the advice of many who would only speak positively: recite these certain Scriptures, pray these certain prayers, and perhaps even travel to meet with a man who had a track record of praying for people who then experienced healing. Often people would write these comments on the blog; some felt like a reprimand, though I believe the words were said out of love and concern for Nette's well-being.

Another approach could be to look only at medical facts. Kidney cancer, kidney removed. Six months later, it shows up in both lungs. From what doctors where telling us, it was now a death sentence since it had spread.

The path we chose to think along was a combination of the two. We held in tension the medical fact—Nette had less than a year to live—while praying for God to do the miraculous. I know we were misunderstood by many who would have hoped for us to only choose "faith" in God. My argument is, we did! We chose to believe no matter the outcome God was with us and, He is good. That choice led to some very, very rich days . . . days filled with incredible life, and staggering amounts of grief. No one lives without one day dying, even when the dying feels incredibly early. If we had only walked in faith, as defined by those who would accept nothing less than physical healing, we would have missed an enormous amount of living. I say that to bring clarity for you as I write about the weeks and months to come.

CHAPTER 11

Freefall

Interleukin (IL 2) had failed; now she had less than a year to live. One day while sitting on the cardiac floor of Northwestern Memorial I began surfing the internet for a destination for a family vacation and for whatever reason I settled on Naples, Florida. It seemed like a beautiful place, and it was on the ocean. As I sat with my laptop open to the Naples webpage, my cell phone rang.

"Hi, Scott. It's Dave." David is Annette's oldest brother who lived almost two hours away. "Scott, there is a man in our church who has a second home. He called to ask if your family would like to use it for a week. It's in Naples, Florida. Is that okay?"

You know, there are times when I just want to drop to my knees and worship. I think I stammered something affirmative through my amazed lips. I literally was looking at the Naples, Florida, website *that* minute. I will tell more about that trip a little later in the story.

August the second. Every year, for the past 16 years, Nette and I had looked forward to August second. It was that day we exchanged words of promise . . . words that as a twenty-one year old, I had no idea what I was saying. Words like: for better . . . for worse . . . in sickness . . . in health. Here we were, on our seventeenth anniversary, sitting on the seventh floor of a hospital in downtown Chicago. Over the years we had spent several anniversaries exploring that beautiful city, along with many other destinations—one of the favorites being Prince Edward Island. Great memories. Now life had delivered us here: seventh floor, cardiac unit. If we held to the doctors' opinions, it would be our last. If not... uncertainty shrouded what Nette's health would be a year away. We talked and talked—and cried. Grief was tangible. I read a quote from Queen Elizabeth not long ago, "The cost of love is grief." When you've opened your heart to another, the thought of not having them is almost indescribable. It's physical. Nurses and other medical staff would come and go as we sat reminiscing, tears streaming down our faces. It wasn't important to hold up any sort of image; we were grieving! Grieving the loss of dreams we shared that had not yet been fulfilled, grieving for our four children who would suffer the loss of their loving mother. Grief—pure, raw, grief. It almost made you want to vomit. Anguish from the very core of who we are as human beings.

Paul wrote in one of his letters that there are times when all we have are wordless sighs and aching groans. That is well said. Jesus had a similar experience before being dragged off to trial. He was so full of grief . . . anguish so intense . . . that he sweated blood. Once again, this "man"—called Christ—informed us how to live. He prayed so hard that He would not have to go through what was in front of Him, but still He submitted. The Bible says He drank the cup all the way to the dregs—you know that nasty stuff at the bottom of your coffee in the morning. All the bitter, disgusting stuff—He drank it all, did it all. We were being asked to do the same; and like Christ, pleaded for another path—anything but this.

Nette was released from the hospital within a day or so following our anniversary. Dr. Stein wanted Nette back within a week to begin a new type of treatment called Torisel. It had very few side effects and promised a certain quality of life while holding the multiplying cells at bay. The trouble was, it was shown to be effective for only six months. At first

Nette was unsure she wanted to do it at all. Her thinking was that if she was going to die anyway, why prolong the agony for a mere six months of living?

Every circumstance is different and each person in that place must make his own decision. Ultimately, Nette had a will to live and even if it was to be just six months, she decided it was worth it. Each time she looked at our four children—especially our four-year old son—she got a fresh will to fight. Lying in bed at night she often cried herself to sleep as we talked of all that she would miss. It was particularly hard thinking of Zach. What memories would he have of Mommy? Would he remember how much he loved to "nuggle" with Mom in the morning and hug so tightly that it seemed he desired to be back inside her skin? We kept our oldest two children, Logan, 16, and Meagan, 14, current, each of them asking to be informed in real time as to what was going on.

A result of that latest news was that Nette became more intentional. She wrote letters to each of the children about her love and dreams for them. Logan voiced his grief that Mom would not be present on mile marker events in life such as graduation, getting married, and the birth of his first child. Not only did Nette write letters, but she also recorded CDs for each one of us; that way, we would always have her voice. She read Karrigan's favorite books and retold many stories an eight-year old never tires of hearing. It took an incredible amount of courage for Nette to be able to do that for our children. If we had only walked in "faith" that God must heal, the kids and I would have been robbed of the lasting gifts Nette was able to leave behind.

Torisel began and initially had some remarkable results. The tumors showed signs of decreasing. If she were to have passed you on the street, you would have had no idea she had less than a year to live. She looked and felt great. One of the dark little pleasures she enjoyed was that if a coughing spell hit, say, in the middle of Wal-Mart where people did not know her and someone offered sympathy for such a bad cough (something like, "Oh dear, you have such a bad cold"), she liked observing their faces turn pale while she explained that she had cancer in both lungs. Dark, yes, but somehow it brought her comic relief.

Yet again, life began to settle into a predictable rhythm. Weekly, Nette went to the local cancer center and received an hour treatment of Torisel. Generally, the side effects wore off within a day or so. Nette even felt well enough to return to some of her regular duties as the pastor's assistant. It was a job she loved and her skills had been missed in the office.

Have you ever heard a speaker try to get the audience motivated to make life changes? They offer a challenge something like, "If you knew you only had six months to live . . ." And then they fill in the blank with whatever the purpose of their speech was. I lived it and know it is almost impossible to do. Even if you knew your expiration date, it is very hard to maintain that level intentionality in all your actions. You do not always speak kindly, you do get hung up on little stuff . . . you're still you. Yeah, you try really hard not to get overly anxious that the house is a mess. You try to remember that taking a walk with the one you love is more important than an empty clothes hamper. It didn't always happen. Nette and I still had disagreements; we didn't always keep in mind we might not have much longer together. Nette still got after the kids; she was still here, she still parented. At times, the kids swiped the "cancer credit card," as we came to call it. Whenever it was advantageous to anyone of them to get his way, he used his cunning skills to get on Mom's good side. In short: we lived life.

Part of living included taking that family vacation to Naples, Florida. A little over a month after the phone call came offering the free lodging; our entire family was on an airplane to the Sunshine State. What a gift! After picking up the rental van, we plugged the address into the G.P.S. The closer we got to the checkered flag marking our final destination, the more excited we became. This house was BEAUTIFUL! When we entered, the kids could not help themselves: "Come look at this," "Oh Mom, look at that!" The property was for sale, so the real estate sheet was placed on the granite counter. It listed for $630,000. Nice! The in-ground, indoor pool—overlooking the golf course with a rock waterfall streaming into the clear warm water—became the kids' hangout. What an amazing gift. God had generously provided this extravagant place—through a man we had never met.

The trip was a "remember when" type of week. I'll explain. I have always enjoyed stories. When I was a boy, we would go to Grampy Shaw's farm on Sunday afternoons. It would not take long before the "remember when" stories started. "'Member when we held Bill and Gary over the pig pen while calling for the swine to come?" That was always a good one. Or, "Remember when Uncle Merle took apart the brand new watch?" . . . On and on they would go.

Creating family stories that bound us all together . . . shared experiences about which the younger generations would never tire of hearing. It was one of those kinds of vacations. I hope to be around the table one day surrounded with grandkids and the stories start something like, "Remember when we rented jet skis in Florida? Dad and Mom made the kids get off and wade through the pounding surf so they could act like juveniles without our screams to 'Slow down!' coming over their shoulder." "Yeah, do you remember Dad spraying salt water over Logan with his jet ski? Loge was momentarily blinded and ran smack into Dad's machine and almost broke Dad's hand." Then someone else chimes in, "How 'bout when Meagan got pulled over by a police boat for speeding in a no-wake zone—we joked they were going to take her to jail . . ." Not very funny to her 13-year old mind. "Remember when the dolphins swam right beside us," Zach might say, everyone recalling how his four-year-old mouth would not stop chattering about it. Karrigan tells her children about the airboat ride through the mangrove swamp filled with gators. It was an excellent vacation. Beaches . . . sunsets . . . walks . . . meals . . . conversations—extravagant! There were moments we almost forgot cancer was part of our vocabulary.

That summer a movie came out staring Jack Nicholson and Morgan Freeman, portraying men who had been given terminal diagnoses. The movie was called *"Bucket List."* The premise was that if you knew you were about to die, you might as well live while you still can. The main characters compiled a list of things they would enjoy and set out to do as many as they possibly could. Nette, not embracing the idea of dying very well, found the movie to be quite compelling. She put together her own bucket list ranging from writing letters to friends to snorkeling in the Caribbean.

Like in the movie, Nette started checking things off. One thing she dreamed of doing was participating in a 5K run. There was one scheduled in the fall, so she and I began working towards that goal. Each morning we got up early and weaved our way through the streets of Ottawa. Ottawa is not large, 18,000 to 20,000, so we knew a lot of people. Often, people would say when they saw Nette running it gave them inspiration to do something they had been putting off. Here was a lady who had less than a year to live, cancer in both lungs, running three-plus miles a day. Some days were better than others. There were times she was so determined to do it, yet her lung capacity could not keep up; she held onto my arm as I kept pace. The assist was enough to keep her pushing towards the next goal. She kept accusing me of changing the stopping point. "Let's keep running till the next stoplight, then we'll stop," I would tell her. When we would arrive at the designated spot, I told her, "I meant the next one." Most times it worked.

Those morning runs were doing more than toning leg muscles and expanding our lungs—they were repairing our relationship as well. It has been only months earlier that

Nette wrestled with whether she needed me in her life or not. Now she asked me to stay by her side so she could pace herself. Our hearts continued to heal. It felt good to have my wife back.

The race was held on a gorgeous mid-October Saturday morning. The buzz of the gathering crowd energized us. A good friend, the pastor of another church in the community, had committed to running alongside Nette and me. I'm sure he could have easily outpaced both of us since he was in great physical shape, but he graciously slowed his pace and matched ours. It was good to have his support. The way the course had been set up, the finish line was on the other side of a gentle curve and a small rise in the path. We could not see the crowd that had amassed along the route leading up to the finish. Friends and family waiting for our return heard Nette was close to completing the race so they pressed their way to the front of the cheering crowd. I'm not sure how we will be ushered into the next life, but what we experienced that day was an incredible metaphor for what it might be like. People were lining the route cheering and yelling out names of those that were still in the race. "Come on—you can make it! Great job . . . you're almost there . . . keep going!" It caused us to forget sore leg muscles and burning lungs. Cheers of the crowd were carrying us to the end. Jubilant tears flowed as hugs and high fives were exchanged. We made it! I know it was only a simple 5K run, just over three miles, but it might as well have been an ascent to the top of Mt. Everest or being awarded the Nobel Prize. She had done it! What a feeling!

The routine was to run every other day. The race was on Saturday, so our plan was to resume running again Monday. It never happened. Nette never was able to run again after that glorious Saturday. Monday, we began the normal routine of walking for a block then easing into a slow jog that finally evened out to a pace of a ten-minute mile. We had run less than a block when pain in her side stopped us. Nette had achieved her goal of completing a 5K and it appeared that it was just in time.

Several items on the list Nette was able to complete without me. She wanted to drive a Cadillac convertible—done. Reconnect with a friend she had lost contact with—check. On and on she worked diligently, trying to do as much as possible while her health continued. The doctor told us that the health she was experiencing today was not an indication of what it might be a month from now. That was sobering and informing: make every minute . . . day . . . week count—no waste.

Annette completed many things on her list without me; there were some, however, we enjoyed together. Snorkeling in Cancun was one of them. Nette intended to make travel plans after she had the first signs of deteriorating health. There was something about doing everything on her list. She wrestled with, what if she did everything and then ended up living for another twenty years? We would have spent money that could have gone for more pressing things—more practical things. The other side of that coin was that, if she didn't live, then everyone loses. We could have lived conservatively and not made the trip to Florida—airfare for all of us, food, rental car, recreation. It was expensive—money I never regret spending.

Here we were making travel plans to Cancun, Mexico. It was such a strange, awkward time. Nette looked as healthy as anyone you might pass at a shopping mall, yet there was this diagnosis of terminal cancer. She felt guilty about traveling, running, hanging out with friends, etc. What would people think? Our friends had worked so hard doing the benefit for our family and now, would they think we were wasting it all? At times her thoughts of what others might think held her hostage. She wouldn't go out of the house, thinking she did not look sick enough to be a cancer patient. It was in this context she did her own internet search and found a great deal on a quick retreat to Cancun—after a lot of persuasion from friends and myself. It was a short three-night/four-day stay, which holds lasting memories. Soon after we were airborne she was glad to be on the journey.

The purpose for our trip was for Nette to be able to snorkel . . . and snorkel we did. As soon as we landed and threw the bags in our room, we began our search for who had the best excursions. We found an excellent one. They were over the top. The van picked us up from the resort first thing in the morning and was scheduled to make several more stops picking others up along the way. No one showed—allowing us to have a personal tour. I am not good enough with words to capture the beauty that is hidden just beneath the waves, stunning beauty that only a small percentage of people will ever see. Nette would later write that her eyebrows were stuck to her hairline because her eyes were taking in such wonders. As we reflected over lunch about what we had seen, Nette reported she had come back to shore changed. She kept repeating over and over to herself as she floated above the coral, "If God can create this world—this world only a handful of people see—I can trust His plan for me." There was comfort in knowing that God is in control of it all.

The month of December flew by, Cancun at the beginning, followed by numerous holiday parties, and finally Christmas. There was such a whirlwind of activity we hardly paid attention to the "C" word. Nette continued the once-a-week treatment of Torisel, and aside from a little fatigue and some nausea, life was fairly manageable. Christmas was bittersweet as we thought of where we had been over the last several months . . . and then thinking ahead into the unknown of the New Year and what it might bring. It does not matter how many times you lay down the notion that we are not in control of life and death . . . it still is a haunting thought to face a holiday that may be your last. As night gave way to Christmas morning, Nette and I lay in bed as torrents of tears flowed. What if it were the last Christmas morning?

What if this young mother would never again hear shrieks of excitement as her children opened long anticipated gifts? I know I wrote about the deep agony of grief earlier . . . but I must mention it again . . . and again. Grief washed over the family in wave after wave as we faced another new awareness. We could only force the stark reality from our mind for so long—there are only so many distractions. The thoughts came as strong as a gale-driven wave slams into the sea wall—a new reality of loss hit. Anyone observing through the frosted window would not—could not— have guessed the underlying feeling of dread holding us in its grip.

January 1, 2009. Health had held fairly well on the new treatment Dr. Stein had prescribed. There were the beginnings of signs letting us know it may not hold much longer. So far this writing has been from my perspective of walking through the "valley of the shadow of death," as David called it in the Psalms. I also want you to hear from Nette's perspective. The following paragraphs were written January 1st as Nette looked toward an uncertain new year.

"I've never been skydiving – don't even want to try – but there is an idea in my mind of what it would be like. I imagine myself to be doing just that as the anticipation builds inside of me, entering this New Year. It's like I'm standing close to the door used to jump, not quite knowing WHEN the altitude is just right. I can't see the pilot's controls so I don't know exactly, but I know that when it comes and the time is ripe for me to freefall out of the plane, I'll be scared. I imagine the view is spectacular and new visions are revealed, but still the heart pounds as every thought of death passes through the mind only put to rest when the parachute opens.

I will begin my freefall shortly – don't know when – but as I contemplate this year, I can foresee the door of the plane opening for the jump – my heart pounds . . .

71

Really, the story I want to share is the story of Abraham. Back in those days, it wasn't unusual for the people to be sacrificing their kids to their gods. Abraham's God had instituted using certain animals as sacrifices. But on one particular day, Abraham heard from God that he was to offer his son as a sacrifice — the son that God had miraculously provided from the dried up old womb of Abe's wife. He'd waited years for this kid. All his hopes were pinned on this kid. God has promised that Abe's descendants would be like the sand of the sea and the stars of the sky. But now God wanted that very son He gave. The Bible says that early next morning they set out, up the mountain, to obey. Usually when I've heard or read this story, I've kept reading until the beautiful part when God shows up, but recently I've gotten a whole new glimpse on it. I've allowed myself to think about Abraham's grief.

It would be inhuman to overlook that this man would have grieved his whole way up the mountain, even through the night, hoping for God to intervene, but willing to continue up the mountain. I've stopped reading sometimes — not letting myself read the ending. Abraham wouldn't have known the ending. He would have just been a man, giving up his son. Grief . . .

That story merged the whole idea of having faith and preparing to die. I'm not afraid to admit that none of the medicines have worked for me that would have bought me years of time. (Scott reminds me often that one of my gifts is my pragmatism). The medicine that is working only buys me six months of time, of which five have been wonderfully spent. We are grieving. Our kids are grieving. We are talking together with a couple of families, weekly, of life as it is now, and life as we prepare for death. We talk of the hope of God's intervention and miracles. We talk words of love and longing.

Abraham's story has given me permission to prepare. Hope yes, but not excluding preparation . . . it's not one camp or the other, reality or faith. It's both. It's given us permission to grieve what will be, unless God intervenes. It's not robbed us of hugs and beauty and love words spoken. It's empowered us to talk openly about God being with us WHILE we are in amazing conversations and insights into one another.

So, if you keep reading, you will see evidence of my preparations to die. It is not because I do not hope. It is because I love the family and friends I will leave behind if I do die. If we prepare but God heals me, we will have walked closely; with no regrets, through a difficult season, and we will praise God together knowing how close we were to death. If we prepare and it is God's purpose not to heal, those around me will have been given permission to grieve and my kids will not be set up for disillusionment with God had we only spoken healing. Even Jesus visiting the towns he did, healed only some. Three of my friends with cancer recently died while hoping until their last breath for a miracle. By living, preparing to die, we all win.

So, 2009? All I can say is that the door to the plane will open when my body stops responding to this medicine, and I will free fall into the arms of God's purposes.

Or, like the story of Abraham, we continue to walk up the mountain, not knowing how God will provide.

My heart pounds."

We were soon to find out the door had already begun to open. Pain in the region of the ribs began to be more and more frequent, breathing more labored, and fatigue set in. All were signs pointing to deteriorating health. Nette was grateful she had not waited, as she had planned on doing, until the first bad doctor's report before booking a snorkeling vacation—it would have never happened.

January was a whirlwind of activity at Nette's work. Since she was the pastor's assistant a large portion of the detail planning for a celebration weekend fell on her desk. Being conscientious, Nette pushed through growing weariness so that everything got completed for the Saturday/Sunday festivities. Long days and late evenings began to take their toll. The weekend went perfectly: power point presentations, annual reports, guest accommodation—all went flawlessly under Nette's guidance.

Monday morning, Nette's energy reserve began to be depleted. Monday night, our family joined our pastor's family and one other single mom with her son for a meal. This had become part of our weekly routine. Our pastor, who held a license in counseling, offered to enter the grieving process with us as we created a safe place for the children to speak about how they were doing. It was the best thing we could have done. Nette's desire was to hold her children as they grieved. Each Monday we came together for a meal then gathered in the living room and entered into the most incredible conversations. Tears freely flowed; teenagers, who often retreat into silence, spoke openly of how great a loss it would be without Mom. Logan confessed of the veneer he had been holding up . . . his rationale was to be strong for his younger siblings by not showing his emotions. Once he spoke it out loud, something inside broke. Meagan wrapped her arms around him as they both wept bitter tears. One of the troubling thoughts in Karrigan's mind was what if Dad married a mean step-mom? The image in her young mind of a stepparent came from Disney's movie *"Parent Trap."* From this classic, Karrigan thought all stepparents sent the children away to boarding school . . . or never let them leave their room. Nette assured her little eight-year-old, "Daddy will choose a good one."

Monday after Monday we were amazed at the rich conversations taking place—things neither Nette nor I had any idea was on our children's minds. Once more, I emphasize that if we had only held onto speaking nothing but healing, we would have been robbed. If we had listened to the voice of critics, it would have robbed the Roix children of memories that will most likely last a lifetime.

As you are reading this memoir of our family's passage I want to say something to you personally. I don't have any idea what you, your children, or anyone close to you is going through. It may not be renal cell carcinoma like the path we walked, but it is every bit as dark. Christ, the one I unashamedly follow, said that in this life— on this planet—there is going to be trouble (I'm paraphrasing). Don't be surprised when the phone rings and there is horrible news pouring from the speaker: Cancer . . . There's been an accident . . . Natural disaster has devastated everything . . . Job cutbacks . . . Spouse wants a divorce . . . on and on and on the list can go. There is unfathomable grief in this life! How excellent is that? If that's the message of this man/God, the hell with it . . . let's get drunk! **It's not!!!** He wasn't done talking: yes, there is trouble — everyone will have his or her share, no one exempt. Money, power, fame . . . nothing insulates humanity from heartache. Jesus did not let those to whom He was talking hang in despair. "Don't be afraid. I have overcome."

I have learned that Jesus was not being braggadocios in telling his followers that He had overcome; He was instructing them to live as He lived. Love—love extravagantly, love those who hurt you; abundantly love. He wasn't talking about the cheap tabloid love that sells at the end of the checkout lane— no, not that. This is true, deep, rich love. If we have that—live that way— we are wealthier than anyone with all the material goods of this earth. I'm not speaking of some ooey–gooey feeling that gets mistaken for love. No, this is much more filling than that. It is knowing first and foremost: *God loves me.* When that went from my head to inside my heart, the deepest part of my understanding, it changed how life looked. I have known it on an intellectual level for most of my life: "Jesus Loves You!" It never meant much until something clicked—HE REALLY DOES LOVE ME. I know it is true because this man of history, called Christ, lived life— just like you and me. His good friend, Lazarus, died; He knows grief. He did not pretend it didn't hurt; He wept. He knows what it feels like to be sexually abused, paraded naked in front of people; yet the story reads like He almost couldn't help Himself as He hung on the Roman cross of execution: "God . . . please . . . FORGIVE THEM!" No, He wasn't bragging. He lived it and invites us to live it too. When I read His words it feels like the wisdom of a gentle father to his child. "Don't be afraid . . . it is going to be okay. I know there are going to be things that happen to you while you live on earth. They happened to Me, too! Listen to Me now: if you do what I showed you, live like I lived, you can make it. And I'm right here to help you."

February 3, 2009. We returned from the Monday night meal and guided conversation around 8:30. We hurried the kids to bed since they all had school the next morning. Nette was ready for a quiet house so she, too, could burrow into her bed and recharge her depleted body. Nette always had the ability to fall asleep quickly. She could be having a conversation one minute and be off in dreamland the next. Such was the case that night. Her sleep was soon interrupted. Unrelenting waves of nausea began to wash over Nette. She could not stop heaving. The constant convulsing of stomach muscles caused the already growing pain in Nette's ribs to be magnified all the more. There is never an easy diagnosis when you have cancer. Normally, it would've been dismissed as a really, really bad flu. Everything in us wanted to believe that. By Thursday, Nette was worn out, the pain great enough that she reluctantly allowed me to take her to the ER. After three liters of fluid and chest x-rays showing signs of pneumonia, doctors determined that Nette needed to be admitted. After several days in the hospital, the attending physician pulled me aside. "I think you need to tell your wife to have the conversations she wants to have."

As much as we may have thought we were making preparations for this moment, the words had the impact of a head-on collision. She had been so healthy; looked so good. Now, suddenly—at least it felt that way—we were being told to begin saying good-bye. The all too familiar feeling of grief's embrace took hold once again. When I looked into the crumpled face of our beautiful eight-year old daughter, knowing there was absolutely nothing I could do to shield her from life's agony, my heart sobbed.

Educated guesses of the team of doctors who had cared for Nette told us she had about eight weeks left. Nette wanted her last days spent in familiar surroundings, not the sterile environment of a hospital. Hospice became involved and transformed a family room holding mountains of memories into a waiting room . . . waiting for the hour when death would overtake life. The days and weeks following Nette's coming home were the most tortured of my life. Hope: Nette just got off her bed and ate a cheeseburger—that must mean . . . ! Despair: Nette needed an injection of pain meds between her regular intervals—that must mean . . . ! Back and forth, back and forth—like the ebb and flow of the ocean; emotions were shredded. Frequently people stopped by the house and by chance saw Nette at one of her better moments; they left proclaiming she was on the path to health. It made me so angry!

What they didn't see, ten minutes after their leaving, was Nette vomiting in a bucket. Tension began building between long-time friends. I became less and less welcoming to requests to drop by. Even in Nette's weakened, drug clouded mind she wanted to be gracious to her guest—only to pay for it moments later.

As if I didn't have enough to wrestle with in my thoughts already, here was one more thing to add to the pile. Everyone had been generous beyond words. Hot meals were brought in every day, more cookies than we could possibly eat, a vehicle, gas, yard work, coffee—anything we needed and some that we didn't, was being attended to. Yet, I felt the need to build a protective cocoon around Nette and our children. To our friends it may have felt like I had become a control freak. It wasn't my intention. My motive was to allow those who were experiencing the greatest loss—Logan, Meagan, Karrigan, and Zachary—to have the most access. If I had allowed the house to fill with friends (and it would have), there would have been nothing left for the kids.

Over the next eight weeks Nette's health could be charted like a declining stock market. Moments—even whole days, there would be signs of improvement. She kept applesauce down for three hours! She is getting up and sitting in a chair! We grasped at anything indicating recovery; the truth was that the trend was decline. Nette was now on constant oxygen and her pain meds increased. Care giving became unmanageable alone. A PICC line had to be re—inserted so medicine could be injected instead of administering pills, which Nette was not able to digest without nausea. The longest space between any of the assortment of medicines was three hours: round the clock, 24/7. The days were checked off by hour intervals. A constant beeping of a cell phone's alarm would alert the next treatment. Momma Margaret took up residence with us and most nights insisted that I rest while her own sleep was disrupted every hour. The agony of grief for this beautiful mother tore at my heart. It's not "supposed" to be this way! Mothers don't watch their youngest child die! Day after day, we watched the invasive cells deteriorate this seemingly healthy body. Once so vibrant, full of life and energy; now just a shell! Skin once stretched over toned muscles now hung like oversized draperies on a frail skeleton. Only five months had passed since this same body had carried Nette across the finish line of a 5K in a respectable thirty-three minutes—it was now a laborious process to go the thirteen feet to the bathroom.

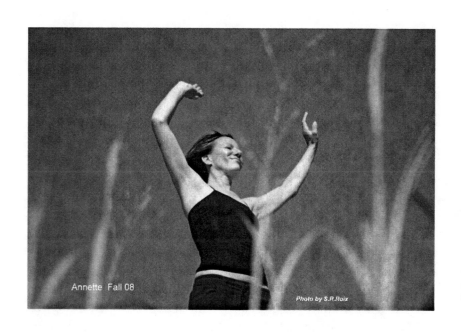

Annette Fall 08

Photo by S.R.Roix

CHAPTER 12

The Struggle Is Over

April 7, 2009. I suppose if a random sampling of people were asked to look back on that date on their day planner or scroll across the days on a Blackberry, there would be any number of responses: Started a new job, took the dog to the vet, changed the oil in the car, 3:30 dentist appointment, or birth of first child. For some it was a highlight in their lives, to others it was just another mundane day stacked on top the heap that compiles our lives. For those of us connected to Annette Kaye Stanfield Roix, it was the pinnacle of grief.

At 8:05 a.m., we were sitting at the kitchen table with cups of coffee as we had done for so many days over the last two months: Margaret, Alice the hospice nurse and incredible friend, and myself. Alice looked across the dining room into the family room where Nette was nestled in her hospital bed. "Scott, you may want to gather the kids, I don't think it will be long," Alice urged. Seven of us assembled around the bed of a well-loved daughter, mother, wife, and friend. The room with which each of us was infinitely familiar . . . became sacred. The moment death overtook life. I leaned over the bedside and whispered the last words into my lover's ear: "Nette, we're all here. We love you. You can go now." Silence, no more struggling—life was over.

Thirty-nine years and a few days is the time Nette spent on this earth. She lived life; she knew pain that accompanies so many, she also knew love. In the end, LOVE WINS. The night before the funeral I stood at the head of the casket and shook over eleven hundred hands. As people passed by, they told how their lives had been affected as a result of knowing Annette. I was humbled and honored to be her husband.

If you recall, I spoke earlier about trouble our relationship had weathered over the last year. Healing had come to us as a couple. The day of Nette's death I knew her love and commitment to me, and mine to her. One of my commitments was I would not leave her. I realize it was only a symbolic act, but it was important for me to do: the night before the funeral I arranged for a couch to be placed in the auditorium in front of the casket. I did not sleep much that night. I paced back and forth before the shell that once was known as Nette. I told her how thankful I was for the seventeen years we had shared; thanked her for the living reminder each time I look at our four children; spoke of dreams that would never be fulfilled. Mostly, though, I just cried. I know I've said it before— a lot— but I say it again: grief was tangible! My whole being grieved. Crying did not seem adequate to express the sorrow that held so tight.

The next day, close friends and family assembled to say our final goodbyes. That is exactly the way it felt. Death is final. No more words, no more anything. It was such a strange new world. Realization was settling in— it's *over*. As I looked on the screen playing scenes of happier times, the thought kept scrolling through my mind, "That was my life . . . that was what I knew . . . that was familiar." Everything going forward is foreign.

God gave me wisdom that day for two things. One was allowing Logan to be one of the men who shouldered the weight of the casket. He honored his mother in that act. The other was letting Zach . . . carry his light saber. There were no parent-of-the-week awards to be given, no pretenses to hold up. If a plastic toy brought a measure of comfort to a child who was looking at Mommy in a casket, well, then, he could carry the sword.

The day was the most surreal experience; it was as if I were an unattached observer. This can't be me . . . can't be my life. I'm a young man—I have young children. No, this can't be true. Only a few weeks had passed since she had looked so full of life. Now she was gone . . . her voice forever silenced. I stood at the curb as the casket was loaded into the hearse to be carried away. I had come as far as I could— promise kept: I would not leave you alone. But now we live in different worlds: Nette in a place of rest from this life struggles, and I . . . remain here.

CHAPTER 13

What's Next, Papa?

The hours . . . days . . . weeks following Nette's death blur in my memory. There was so much to attend to, so many things I was not accustomed to doing, now my sole responsibility. One thing I knew: I wanted to go home—home to my family. I had been gone from my parents and sister in Maine for almost two decades and longed to feel the strength of their love surrounding me in my season of immense grief. Christ Community Church had been over the top in their support for the Roix family—nothing left out; they had attended to all our needs . . . a beautiful sacrifice of love.

Still . . . I longed to rest in my father's home. The kids and I made the grueling twenty-plus hour drive retracing routes we had traveled many times over the years. From the moment of our arrival, Nana (my mom), took over! It had been such an intense season of being caregiver, grieving husband, guiding father to hurting children— I had had no time to quiet my mind and pray my prayers. My parents insisted I take their car and spend the day at one of my favorite places along Maine's coast. What a gift! The day was spectacular—driving a Jaguar along coastal routes, top open, praying prayers from the core of my soul. I found my way to a familiar rock and spent the day talking to God. I remember how sunny it had been inland as I drove to the coast, but as I sat at the ocean's edge, dense fog rolled in concealing everything except for a few yards in front of my seat. It was so appropriate. The rest of the world was enjoying the warm sun, and there I was . . . alone . . . in the fog. Uncertainty surrounding my life, "What's next, Papa?" became my mantra.

Nature instructs us about the character of the Creator. It was as if I had a front row seat to the object lesson with which He presented me that day. Tons of crashing waves pounded the rock, as they have done for centuries. The rock remained unmoved . . . unshaken . . . unfazed by the severity of each blow delivered by the force of the mighty ocean. My hope, my faith was set firmly on the Rock. He is unmovable! He is not fazed with the severity of life! He, being God— not just any god—no, the One and Only living God of all Creation, He has absorbed pounding waves of grief and loss and turmoil of the human existence since the beginning of time. The density of the fog may have been disorienting to me, but not to Him. He knew exactly where I was . . . known exactly how to navigate the treacherous landscape. And not only make it through, but make it through stronger than when we began the journey. I believe the choice that leads to life, amazing life, is placing trust in God. Trust—He wants to participate in our life journey. Trust— He is good. Trust—He will guide us, when we let Him. There are days when the sun shines brilliantly overhead, all is well; He is the source of that generous gift. But then, there are days when all we have is dense fog and pounding waves—it is a lot harder to trust in that hostile environment. My tendency is to run helter-skelter, retracing my steps back to the sunshine. Life is not like that, though. We cannot relive our days; time marches relentlessly forward.

So many details have flooded my thoughts as I have written about our family's passage. I hit the major ones. There are things I need to tell you as I finish. I would not have wanted to walk through any of that alone. Our family was immersed with extravagant love. I hope I am forever changed in how I live life and give generously to those who are hurting. God has become more real than I ever could imagine. Not a distant, angry Being who I'm sure must be disappointed in me; He loves me. The book, called the Bible, is alive—no longer a religious task to be checked off. It is much, much more than that. It instructs how to live; it's for today. When I started believing *"God so loved the world that He gave His only Son,"* I realized that son, Jesus, experienced everything we have to live through . . . and He made it. When I transitioned from thinking it was a theory, just a nice religious story, to embracing it as true . . . hope blossomed.

Life is incredibly short. Just a wisp of smoke; here for a moment, then vanished. Youth offers the illusion that life goes on and on . . . it doesn't. I can waste a day here and there making little difference in the grand scope of things, but if I compile too many of those days . . . soon I have squandered the most expensive gift I ever received. Why was I ever born if I walk through life asleep? There will only ever be one of me in the history of the universe—only one of you, one person who does life exactly like you. What contribution to mankind can be made while we exist in this world? What expression of God can be shown in stunning beauty through every individual life lived with abandon for Him? Why carry around the baggage of mistrust and hatred that characterizes so much of our world? Why curse God? Why turn to substances that medicate with the illusion of making the pain stop? God is the One Who knows how to live . . . really live.

Have faith; so you look ridiculous—so what? Like I wrote in the beginning, stories recorded centuries ago about a variety of people—they looked nuts, but they believed . . . believed God was leading their life—and each of them lived an incredible story. Moses, for example, if he had not acted on what God told him, even though it seemed like an impossible task, he never would have experienced standing on top of a mountain, face to face with God. He would have died alone in the desert tending sheep. There is nothing wrong with being alone, tending sheep, in a desert . . . except he was born for more than that. That stirs me. Many times, fear has kept me from going the direction I was meant to go—fear of what others would say or think, fear of failing. Even though the path looks uncertain—each step an act of trust in a God I cannot see—I now know He is good, and He is with those who trust Him.

CHAPTER 14

Transition

I read multiple books following the death of Annette trying to gain some perspective on my new circumstances. The year and a half leading up to her passing was the most emotionally charged time I had ever lived through and had left me disoriented. One thing I knew: I had enjoyed being married. Almost everything I read about men who had lost their spouses at a young age indicated that most remarried soon after. Raising four children without someone to help was not very appealing and I missed having a companion to do life with. Within ten months of Annette's death, I remarried to a lady I met through E-harmony named Gina.

I had been talking to my mother throughout the whole process as she always wanted to know if I had found someone I might be interested in. I had made the stipulation that four children were plenty; whomever I met would need to be satisfied with that and not want any more. A short time after Gina and I had been dating I phoned my Mom to tell her about this beautiful lady. Mom wanted all the details, something like women do when a baby is born; they need to know the stats. So I filled her in with the highlights I knew up to that point of our relationship. "Well, does she have or want children?" It was the one piece of info I had been trying to avoid telling her. "Mom, you may want to find a chair for a moment" was my reply. "Gina has **FIVE** children!" Her response was one of shock. The grandchildren count almost doubled . . . instantly.

My decision to remarry so soon was not received well among the community of which I had been a part for many years. In no way did I mean it as disrespect to Annette or to the years that we had shared. The fact was that she was no longer here. I will never forget her impact on my life and the gift she bore of four incredible children. In the marriage vows that I wrote to Gina I stated that she was my choice for the next part of life's journey. Annette had helped to shape who I had become as a man for almost twenty years. Life had brought me to a new place with a new companion who continues to mold who I am becoming.

In that season of transition I chose to sell our home in Ottawa and move to the shore of Lake Michigan in southeast Wisconsin with my new bride and our nine children. The move was particularly hard on my two teenagers. I will forever be grateful that they did not rebel but chose to make the difficult relocation trusting that I knew what I was doing. It was in that climate of change that I closed Community Electric Co. and chose not to obtain an electrical license in my new setting. Instead, I began to put to use my years of training in Biblical studies by volunteering as chaplain at the local hospital . . . which has led to a paid position. It is a privilege to sit with those who are hurting and share the hope that God has given to me.

Shortly after returning from our honeymoon I found myself walking along the shore of Lake Michigan. It has become one of my favorite places for solitude where I can clear my thoughts and pray my prayers. The following is an account of that walk which became the catalyst for writing of this book:

I Will Do It

I was on the ground, under a tree, in the middle of a busy park . . . *crying*. I had heard from God. March 18, 2010, was an absolutely beautiful, late-winter day. The sun shone brilliantly as a breeze shimmered across the sparkling water. That day, I heard from the Creator, the One Who had spoken all of it into being, the God Who maintains order, and the One Who causes seasons to cycle without end. It is that God Who spoke to me.

Here is a glimpse into my thoughts that led up to that day's conversation. I had been reading in Genesis about the hall-of-famer, Abraham. This man had an unbelievable confidence in God. God's response to Abraham's faith was, "I am going to bless you; I am going to bless you indeed." I could hear the joy in God's voice as He prepared and poured out His blessing on the one who so completely trusted in Him. It was to this passage that my thoughts turned as I sat beside the great lake.

I could not concentrate on the task I had intended to do, so I exited the car to walk the path along the shore. As I set out, I told God *I* would talk going one way, and asked for *Him* to speak as I made my way back. Prayer poured out of me as I began taking the first few steps. I told God of my fears and longings; I told Him how I was so unsure of where I was at this point in my life. I did believe an unseen God was ordering my steps. All my hopes and dreams were in one basket—*There is a God who knows and cares where I am (we are) personally.* These were the paths of thought that my prayers followed.

That day was just delicious. After the cold and snow and bareness of winter, this was a day that pointed to the coming of a new season. I walked and prayed for a long time. Finally, with nothing left to say, I turned to make my way back. I closed my mouth and waited for God's response.

I walked for about two football-field lengths—*nothing*. "OH GREAT! This is pretty much a one-sided conversation." I still desired to keep my thoughts turned to God, so I began to think on the Scripture I had read earlier in the day. Well, I got stuck on one phrase: " . . . Abraham fell on his face and worshiped."

Now, exactly how *do* we hear from God? That is an ongoing question for me. Yet, I had the feeling that the Spirit was saying, *"Lie down."* Bill Cosby has a comedy routine: Noah gets a message from God telling him to build a boat because there is going to be a flood. Noah responds, "YEAH, RIGHT!" That was pretty much my feeling: "Yeah right, like I am going to lie down on this public path with . . . a LOT of people enjoying the day." So . . . I just kept walking . . . with the persistent thought, *"Lie down."*

Okay, so, being a curious guy by nature, I decided I had better do it or I might miss out on something if this was, indeed, God. Just ahead I saw a little knoll with a lone tree on it. Someone lying under tree . . . on a hill . . . on a day like this . . . might not appear *too* odd. Leaving the path, I found a spot that looked dry and I stretched out, looking up at an endless blue sky. Instantly, a familiar thought came to me, *"He makes me to lie down."* Well, having grown up in church my whole life, my mind automatically finished the sentence from the famous Psalm: *"He makes me lie down . . . and He restores my soul."*

"Oh, I get it!" I had not yet understood what He was doing in my life. "Why wasn't anything opening up for me to do?" As I lay there thinking of the last two years of my life, His Spirit spoke to my spirit and let me know, "Scott, I am restoring your soul." He loved me so much that He had been allowing me time to catch my breath. I dwelt on that as I rested beneath the tree, gazing through branches that had not yet budded.

The next thing the Spirit spoke to me was, "I WILL DO IT." Something clicked as I lay there looking up through that tree. Spring was about to begin to bring buds. Nothing could stop spring. Nothing! There was not a force big enough to stop the next season from happening. "I WILL DO IT!" After getting back into my car, I picked up the *Message* version of the Bible and read, "*You bedded me down in lush meadows . . . you let me catch my breath . . . and sent me in the right direction.*" Is that what God had been doing? Oh, wow! That was His word to me, "Scott, catch your breath . . . things are about to bud and a new season is going to bring fruit. I, the God Who created all that is, *I* will do it."

Tears of joy ran down my cheeks as I realized Who it was that had spoken to me: GOD . . . *my* GOD . . . the One Who loves and cares for me. Like Abraham, I fell to the ground—and worshiped.

I ask with eagerness . . .

"What's next, Papa?"

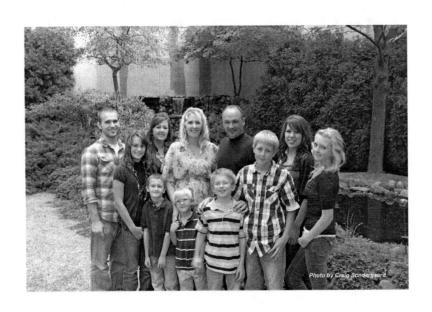

Photo by Craig Sondergaard

CPSIA information can be obtained at www.ICGtesting.com
Printed in the USA
LVOW112128091111

254305LV00001B/175/P